Mutism

Yvan Lebrun, PhD

Professor of Neurolinguistics,
Vrije Universiteit Brussel

W

Whurr Publishers Ltd
London and New Jersey

Whurr Publishers Ltd
19b Compton Terrace
London N1 2UN
England

First published 1990
Reprinted 1990

British Library Cataloguing in Publication Data

Lebrun, Yvan
  Mutism.
  1. Man. Speech disorders
  I. Title
  616.855

ISBN 1-870332-55-5

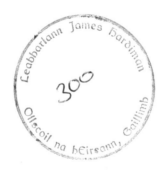

Laserset by Scribe Design, Gillingham, Kent
Printed in Great Britain by Athenaeum Press, Newcastle upon Tyne

General preface

This series focusses upon disorders of speech, language and communication, bringing together the techniques of analysis, assessment and treatment which are pertinent to the area. It aims to cover cognitive, linguistic, social and educational aspects of language disability, and therefore has relevance within a number of disciplines. These include speech therapy, the education of children and adults with special needs, teachers of the deaf, teachers of English as a second language and of foreign languages, and educational and clinical psychology. The research and clinical findings from these various areas can usefully inform one another and, therefore, we hope one of the main functions of this series will be to put people within one profession in touch with developments in another. Thus, it is our editorial policy to ask authors to consider the implications of their findings for professions outside of their own and for fields with which they have not been primarily concerned. We hope to engender an integrated approach to theory and practice and to provide a much-needed emphasis on the description and analysis of language as such, as well as on the provison of specific techniques of therapy, remediation and rehabilitation.

Whilst it has been our aim to restrict the series to the study of language disability, its scope goes considerably beyond this. Many previously neglected topics have been included where these seem to benefit from contemporary research in linguistics, psychology, medicine, sociology, education and English studies. Each volume puts its subject matter in perspective and provides an introductory slant to its presentation. In this way we hope to provide specialized study which can be used as texts for components of teaching courses at undergraduate and postgraduate levels, as well as material directly applicable to the needs of professional workers.

David Crystal
Ruth Lesser
Margaret Snowling

Preface

Several people have helped me write this book – encouraging me to pursue the study of mutism, providing references or reviewing the manuscript. Two of them have been particularly helpful and these are Chantal Leleux and Françoise Devreux. They have both been co-workers with me for many years and we have written a number of papers together. In this book, Chantal has helped me track down much of the literature used and Françoise has assisted me in gathering data; she has also helped me realise how telling silence can be. I am happy to dedicate this book to the two of them.

Y. Lebrun 1989

Contents

General preface   v

Preface   vii

Prologue   1

Chapter 1   5

The psychology of silence

Silence in the Western World
Silence in the monastery
Dumbness

Chapter 2   11

The syndrome of mutism: Introduction

Mutism
 Degree of intentionality
Functional *vs* organic mutism

Chapter 3   15

The syndrome of mutism: Functional mutism

Selective mutism
    In children with normal command of language
    In children with language delay
    In adults
Total mutism
    In individuals with normal language development
    In individuals with underdeveloped language skills
Conclusions

Chapter 4   59

The syndrome of mutism: Organic mutism

Introductory remarks
  The notion of organicity
  Types of organic mutism
Mutism of peripheral origin
  Laryngectomy
  Glossectomy
  Congenital malformations of the vocal tract
  Deaf–muteness
Developmental mutism of central origin
  Cerebral palsy
  Developmental motor aphasia
  Developmental speech apraxia
Acquired mutism of central origin
  Pseudobulbar palsy
  Opercular syndrome
  Mutism associated with a pyramidal hemisyndrome
  Affections of the motor neurones
  Aphasic mutism
  Locked-in syndrome
  Akinetic mutism
  Mutism following surgery in the fossa posterior
  Parkinsonism
  Commissurotomy
  Speech arrests
  Speech apraxia
Conclusions

Epilogue   **105**

References   **107**

Index (Author)   **117**

Index (Subject)   **121**

Prologue

Although mutism is alluded to in many publications and although there are numerous reports of individual cases of mutism, no monograph seems to exist that surveys the various forms of mutism and highlights the similitudes and dissemblances between them. The present study is an attempt to fill this gap.

In this book the word 'mutism' is used to denote a condition in which there is no, or very little, oral–verbal expression, whilst comprehension of speech (and possibly also of written language) is normal or at least at a considerably higher level than oral–verbal output.

The study is based primarily on clinical reports, but it also resorts to literary examples when these may help throw light on the problem. This applies particularly to mutism of psychological origin. Great writers have an insight into the human psyche, and their creations are often beautifully illustrative of behaviours that are of interest to the clinician.

Throughout the study a clinical–semiological approach is used, which attaches great importance to symptomatology, analyses symptoms carefully, studies their nature, occurrence and accompaniments, and on the basis of this analysis endeavours to single out syndromes. It also develops criteria for the differential diagnosis of the various syndromes and tries to understand the pathogenesis of each of the nosological entities it has identified. Finally, it reflects on ways of improving the conditions it has described.

The method is applied here to the study of mutism. On the basis of the observable symptoms the various forms of mutism are identified and classified, and an attempt is made to understand their respective pathophysiologies. Then therapeutic possibilities are discussed.

This approach is used because it is believed that only careful observation of the mute subject's behaviour can lead to an understanding of his condition. As Altshuler, Cummings and Mills (1987) put it, 'there is no substitute for a thorough evaluation guided by knowledge of the

1

differential diagnosis and continued observation until a diagnosis can be confirmed. Only then will the silent patient yield his or her secret'.

Detailed analysis of the symptoms also seems to be a prerequisite for an adequate typology of the forms of mutism. Confusion in classification and terminology can only be avoided if the various features of the diseases under consideration are carefully studied. Joseph Babinski (1904) quite rightly warned that diagnostic errors are often due to imperfect semiotics. He accordingly urged his students to always pay great attention to symptomatology.

Careful examination of the patient's symptoms makes correct classification of his condition possible and at the same time provides an insight into its pathogenesis. This insight in turn generates ideas for therapy. Indeed, in the absence of correct diagnosis, prognosis is likely to be erroneous, and treatment misdirected.

The clinical–semiological approach is sometimes disparagingly called a pigeon-holing method and reproached for failing to develop a unitary model of the conditions studied. However, unitary models all too often blur significant differences and group together affections which are, in fact, dissimilar (Lebrun and Devreux, 1984).

It is not for the botanist to decide how many families, genera and species should exist – taxonomy is determined by nature and reflects the observable botanical reality. Similarly, the number and nature of the syndromes in language pathology should be dictated not by clinicians, but by clinical observations.

Therefore, the present study endeavours to clearly distinguish between the various sorts of mutism and to identify the clinical syndromes of which mutism can be a component. It also strives, whenever possible, to uncover the pathophysiology of mutism and, finally, it offers therapeutic considerations.

Although using a clinical–semiological methodology, this study does not deal exclusively with pathology. A number of behaviours are examined which occur in people considered normal and healthy – this results from the fact that mutism runs the whole gamut of conditions from completely deliberate to semi-voluntary to totally unintentional.

Mutism can be observed in people whose silence is the result of a considered decision and can be broken as soon as the subject chooses to do so. In some, mutism is associated with psychological problems and does not appear to be fully intentional whereas, in others, speechlessness is the consequence of organic damage to the central nervous system and is completely involuntary.

Speech suppression may therefore be a reasoned behaviour which is adopted with a clear objective in mind and has nothing deviant about it. At other times, it is far less rational and creates a number of social and relational problems which may make intervention desirable. Finally, it may be a completely pathological condition that has to be combated for the benefit of those afflicted.

The limits between these broad categories are not always clear and there are a number of borderline cases. It follows that it is not always easy to determine when mutism ceases to be normal and becomes pathological. Accordingly, it is probably better to take every aspect of mutism into consideration rather than to decide more or less arbitrarily where to halt the investigation.

Another reason why mutism in normal subjects needs to be envisaged here is that the value which is generally attached to silence may play a part in the genesis of functional mutism – the latter being one of the forms pathological mutism can take. The fact that silence is often prized in our society may not be irrelevant to the understanding of speech suspension such as that observed in some people with psychological problems. Consequently this book opens with a chapter on the psychology of silence.

An honest effort has been made to offer an exhaustive survey of the various forms of mutism. However, such an endeavour was bound to remain unsuccessful. How could one individual possibly be aware of all the circumstances under which mutism can manifest itself, or of all the syndromes of which it can be a component? The pathology is so complex, so variegated and at times so unpredictable that it will always outwit pathologists. The present survey, therefore, could not be but incomplete.

Also, the author has no experience of language pathology outside the Western World. Accordingly, only the values of silence in Western civilisation are considered and only forms of mutism as they may be observed in Occidentals are studied. Observations made in the Orient are used only occasionally and in as much as they accord with what has been found in Westerners.

Chapter 1
The Psychology of
Silence

Silence in the Western World

A positive value is often attached to silence in Western civilisation. Indeed, silence is frequently considered to be superior to speech. It is said to be golden whilst speech is only silver. As Jewish writings state: 'If a word be worth one shekel, silence is worth two.'

The Bible praises those who can hold their peace: 'He that refraineth his lips is wise' (Proverbs 10: 19). Another biblical proverb (Proverbs 17: 28) states: 'Even a fool, when he holdeth his speech, is counted wise; and he that shutteth his lips is esteemed a man of understanding.' Ecclesiastes (5: 2) accordingly recommends: 'Be not rash with thy mouth ... (and) let thy words be few, for ... a fool's voice is known by multitude of words.'

The warnings of the Old Testament were echoed in early Christian times by Boetius, who wrote in *De Consolatione Philosophiae*: 'Si tacuisses, philosophus mansisses', i.e. 'If you had kept silent, you would have remained a philosopher, i.e. you would have been considered a wise man.'

What remains tacit is often considered to be better or stronger than what is overtly stated. The unexpressed is felt to be more powerful, more momentous or more weighty than what is uttered. For instance, what goes unsaid between lovers is thought to be more important than what is actually expressed. In love, silence is more eloquent than speech. Thomas Campion said: 'Love's silence doth all speech confute.' Lovers feel at times so close that they need no words to communicate. They are one and enjoy their oneness in silence.

A real great love cannot be put into words; neither can a deep sorrow. Great pains too are mute, and in the presence of profound grief silence is often felt more appropriate than speech. When Job's three friends saw his immense affliction, they 'sat down with him upon the ground seven days and seven nights, and none spake a word to him: for they saw that his grief was very great' (Job 2: 13).

5

Talkativeness, the opposite of silence, is generally considered to be a weakness, and garrulity a fault. He who speaks much exposes himself, betrays himself. As it is written in the Scriptures: 'A fool is full of words' (Ecclesiastes 10:14).

Talking is giving away, losing or rushing headlong into danger. 'He that keepeth his mouth keepeth his life; but he that opens wide his lips shall have destruction' (Proverbs 13:3). Sapience grows in and through silence. As Bacon put it 'Silence is like sleep: it refreshes wisdom' (*Novum Organum*). This is echoed in a popular rhyme:

> There was an old owl who lived in a tree
> And the more he heard the less said he
> And the less he said the more he heard
> Now wasn't he a wise old bird

Silence is also a sign of fortitude. In face of adversity it is braver and nobler to keep silent than to protest or to complain. In front of his judges Jesus kept his own counsel (Matthew 27:12; Mark 15:5; Luke 23:9; John 19:9). At the end of Alfred de Vigny's poem 'La Mort du Loup' ('The Wolf's Death'), the wolf, mortally wounded by the hunter, dies stoically without a howl, reminding the poet that under adverse circumstances silence is the highest virtue: 'Seul le silence est grand, tout le reste est faiblesses.' Swinburne agreed: 'Silence is most noble till the end' (in 'Atalanta in Calydon'). Indeed, as Carlyle put it, 'speech is of time, silence is of eternity' ('Sartor Resartus'). This is probably the reason why a period of silence is observed when the dead are remembered during a ceremony.

Silence, however, is associated not only with death but also with life and creation. According to the French poet Paul Valéry, great works of art are often born out of patience and silence. In the artist, every atom of silence bears the promise of a ripe fruit.

Silence is also ascribed with having redemptive power. For instance, in one of the German folk tales recorded by Jacob and Wilhelm Grimm and called 'The Twelve Brothers', a young girl accidentally causes her 12 brothers to be changed into ravens. She is instructed by an old woman that her brothers will recover their human shapes if she remains completely silent for seven full years. At the risk of her life the courageous girl performs this feat and her obstinate silence rescues her siblings.

This story has a variant, which was equally recorded by the Grimms under the title of 'The Six Swans'. In this variant, six brothers are changed into swans following a curse by their own father. They regain their human shapes after their sister has deliberately remained silent for 6 years.

Silence may be the price that has to be paid to gain somebody's favour. There is no dearth of literary works in which a woman imposes a long silence (sometimes of several years' duration) on a man to test his feelings towards her. Through abstinence from speech the lover proves his passion and wins his sweetheart's favours.

There are also various comedies in which one character gets the better of another by keeping silent for longer.

Although it is the opposite of speech, silence may also be a form of communication. As the saying goes, 'it is not the case that a man who is silent says nothing'. Silence sometimes imparts as much, if not more, than speech. Cicero in his harangue against Catilina, said, 'Cum tacent, clamant' (their silence is a cry).

Silence is at times more pregnant than words. A silent retort may be more effective than a loud rejoinder.

Not infrequently silence is taken as giving consent: 'Qui tacet, consentire videtur' (he who keeps silent is considered to agree).

But silence may also mean dissent or disapproval. In Vercors's novel *Le Silence de la Mer (The Silence of the Sea)*, the two main characters refrain from talking to the German officer who has been billeted on them. Their muteness conveys their objection to the presence of an enemy in their house. It is a form of passive resistance.

Silence in the Monastery

A number of religious orders require that their members should remain silent at certains times of the day or in certain places. For instance, in many monastic communities the monks are not allowed to speak after night song or night examen. The great stillness of the night should not be disturbed by any noise.

In some monasteries, no verbal exchanges are permitted in the cloister, the church and the refectory.

In particular St Benedict imposed silence on his disciples, reminding them that the Scriptures have repeatedly warned against talking too much. 'Whoso keepeth his mouth and his tongue keepeth his soul from troubles' (Proverbs 21:23), for 'in the multitude of words there wanteth not sin' (Proverbs 10:19).

Silence is the source of all good and the father of all pious thoughts. It engenders every virtue. On the contrary, speech can easily become pernicious. All too often it degenerates into idle chit-chat, which diverts the soul from higher, more legitimate concerns.

God himself is silence. His perfection is infinite and above language. It is ineffable. On the day of the last judgment the souls of the righteous will be united with God in complete, perfect stillness.

Silence in the convent is thought to favour meditation and to enhance devotion. Indeed, it is often considered a prerequisite of religious life.

Silence is necessary for recollection and spiritual growth. Only people living in silence can really enjoy the grace of God, only they can hear the voice of the Lord. Monastics therefore ought to eagerly cultivate the quiet inner attentiveness of silence.

In some orders, silence is held to be the foundation of cloistral life. Monks and nuns should refrain from speaking whenever possible. If they feel it necessary to communicate verbally, they should restrict themselves to short utterances and speak in a soft voice. In some religious communities, sign language is used in order not to break the holy silence.

Monks and nuns who refrain from speaking with people can better communicate with God. Silence enables them to grow in union with the Almighty. It is only by immersing themselves in silence that cloisterers can meet the Lord and achieve the 'unio mystica'. Silence forms a spiritual cell which, together with the physical cell, isolates them from the world's turmoil and opens their souls to the divinity.

The dialogue with God is itself silent, for the words of the language cannot adequately express the contents of the communication with the Almighty. The Lord can only be reached through silent contemplation. 'Holy desire prays, even though the tongue is silent', as St Augustine put it. Ecstasy proceeds from prolonged devoted silence, which is therefore more important than theology.

Language is inadequate to make revelation communicable. There is a tragic, unbridgeable gap between what is apprehended and what is said. With all his eloquence Aaron was unable to convey Moses's divine experience, as Schönberg's opera so dramatically shows.

Also, because it is self-expression, speech tends to draw the attention to the speaker, and this runs counter to the monastic ideal of humility. Speech should therefore be restrained, in a spirit of mortification and self-denial.

However, taciturnity is not easy to acquire. The rule of silence is hard to heed, for the tongue, this 'inquietum malum', this disturbing goblin, always tries to interfere. Cloisterers therefore should pray with the psalmist: 'Set a watch, O Lord, before my mouth; keep the door of my lips' (Psalm 141: 3). In their effort to hold their peace they should remember Jesus Christ who did not teach until he was thirty and kept silent in front of his judges.

Although Western civilisation generally values silence, there are situations where people are not supposed to hold their peace. For instance, if they do not happen to know the answer to a question they have just been asked, they ought to acknowledge their ignorance verbally and possibly to apologise for it. If someone on the street comes up to you and asks you what time it is, he expects you to say something even if you have no watch and do not have the faintest idea of what the time is. If you simply continue your way silently, your behaviour will be considered rude and be resented.

Also, in a conversation between two partners, if one of them is taking a long turn, the other generally is expected to signal from time to time that he is still with the speaker, that he keeps listening to him and continues to follow his recounting. These signals are usually short words or interjections. Indeed, they may be mere grunts. Occasionally a nod or a movement of the brows will be used instead of a vocal sign.

Total silence on the part of the listener is ordinarily interpreted as a lack of interest or of comprehension, except when the difference in social status is great between the speaker and the listener. A principal reprimanding a pupil will generally not expect verbal or vocal signals from the pupil, unless he asks him a question. But when peers are in conversation, the listener is supposed to indicate from time to time his sustained interest when the speaker takes a long turn. Failing to do so will generally disquieten the speaker who may interrupt his story to make sure the listener is still with him. This is particularly so when the conversation takes place over the telephone and the speaker cannot see the listener.

Silence, then, appears to be somewhat ambivalent in Western society. Whilst generally considered to be a commendable behaviour, it may at times be felt to be inappropriate or boorish. Although the form of silence does not vary, the interpretation it is given does according to the social context in which it occurs.

Dumbness

Whilst self-imposed silence is often praised and is frequently considered a virtue worth practising, dumbness, i.e. involuntary muteness, is usually regarded as a great disadvantage, if not as an evil.

In the past mutes were thought to be possessed by the devil. To render them verbal, the demon had to be driven out of them. The Gospels report that Jesus cured several mutes by exorcising them. For instance, Luke relates that Christ cured a dumb man by 'casting out the devil . . . When the devil was gone out, the dumb spake' (Luke 11:14).

Dumbness may also be a punishment inflicted by the divinity on a mortal for disbelief or misbehaviour. For instance, the Gospel according to Luke (1:11–64) relates that Zacharias could not believe the Archangel Gabriel when the latter told him that his wife Elizabeth would bear him a son. 'I am an old man and my wife well stricken in years', Zacharias said. Gabriel retorted: 'Behold, thou shall be dumb, and not be able to speak, until the day that these things shall be performed, because thou believest not my words.' And Zacharias lost his power of speech.

When his son was born, Zacharias was still unable to talk. The neighbours asked him how he wanted the child to be called. In writing Zacharias bade them to call him John. After that, 'his mouth was open immediately, and his tongue loosed, and he spake, and praised God'.

Similarly, in a German folk tale called 'Mary's Child' and recorded by the

Grimms, the Blessed Virgin strikes a girl dumb because she has trespassed against a rule and refuses to admit her guilt. When the girl finally recognises that she has sinned, she recovers her power of speech.

Western civilisation, then, contrasts silence with speechlessness. Whilst the former is generally valued, the latter is held to be evil. The former is a merit worthy of praise, the latter a fault or a defect that should be combated. Silence opens a man's soul to God, muteness shuts him off from society. Silence is dignified whereas dumbness is deviant. This duality should probably be borne in mind when the syndrome of mutism is approached.

Chapter 2
The Syndrome of
Mutism: Introduction

Mutism

As stated in the Prologue, the term 'mutism' is used in this book to denote a condition in which there is no, or very little, oral–verbal expression, whereas comprehension of speech (and possibly also of written language) is normal or at least at a considerably higher level than expressive speech. It is precisely this large discrepancy between the non-existent or very scanty oral–verbal output and the normal or nearly normal receptive abilities that is characteristic of mutism.

Mutism does not necessarily mean the total absence of sounds produced with the vocal tract. Mute people may make noises either deliberately in attempts to communicate or spontaneously in reaction to various stimuli, e.g. pain. But these noises are not speech sounds. Mutism thus refers to the absence of articulate speech.

Also mutism does not imply total lack of self-expression. Mute individuals may use non-vocal systems of communication. In fact, if literate, they often resort to writing.

Degree of Intentionality

At times, mutism is totally deliberate. For instance, when a prisoner resolves not to answer the questions of those who have captured him, his silence is completely voluntary. He could speak, but for specific reasons decides to stand mute instead. If he is a soldier, he may make no answer because he does not want to provide the enemy with strategic information. If he is a partisan, he may keep silent in order not to betray his family or friends. At times, he will heroically resist torture applied to make him speak.

When someone is arrested by the police, he may refuse to speak in the absence of his lawyer. In some countries, the accused may decline to answer a question if he feels that his answer is likely to aggravate his case.

In these various instances, silence is deliberate. For some specific and considered reason, the subject decides not to speak. Generally this type of silence is observed during examination or questioning and is maintained only as long as the interrogation lasts. The subject usually refuses not only to speak but also to write. However, occasionally someone who is questioned by the police may give in writing a piece of information which he is not willing to give orally.

Silence may also be totally involuntary. For instance, following brain damage, a patient may be unable to express himself orally. He would like to communicate verbally but cannot. An organic lesion prevents him from speaking. In such a case, the subject has not decided to keep silent. He is speechless in spite of himself.

The cause of unintentional mutism is not always organic. Panic or stage fright may render a person temporarily unable to speak. 'Lingua haeret metu' (the tongue gets stuck under the influence of fear), was written by a Latin poet. Emotion too can be dumbfounding.

Silence may therefore be fully deliberate or, on the contrary, completely involuntary. Between these two extremes there are many intermediate stages where the degree of intentionality is less easy to ascertain. Individuals who keep silent in certain places or in the presence of certain people may be experiencing a psychological inhibition which renders their so-called selective mutism less voluntary than it might seem at first sight. On the other hand, psychological factors may aggravate an organically based speech impairment and turn it into complete mutism, i.e. a person who has verbal difficulties may, because of these difficulties, maintain complete silence, although he actually could have spoken a little. Alternatively he may refrain from using the little speech that he has left because of the secondary benefits which he can derive from the total absence of verbal output.

In the aetiology of mutism various motivational factors may play a role. Indeed, the degree of intentionality may vary from case to case and may at times be difficult to assess accurately.

Functional vs Organic Mutism

In clinical practice, a distinction is made between functional (or psychogenic) and organic mutism. The diagnostic label 'functional (or psychogenic) mutism' is used when the individual gives evidence that he can speak but keeps silent under certain circumstances or in the presence of certain people. The label is also used when speech is suppressed, although on examination the peripheral speech organs appear normal and no central lesion can be discovered that would reasonably account for the absence of oral–verbal expression.

On the contrary, 'organic mutism' is spoken of when there is an organic lesion that can reasonably be made responsible for the speechlessness.

Useful as it is, the distinction between functional and organic mutism is not absolute. If functional mutism is omnipresent (as in the case with so-called 'hysterical mutism') and lasts for a long time, it may result in an inability to produce speech which is similar in its effects to some form of organic mutism. Conversely, mutism which is initially of organic origin may be compounded or maintained by secondary psychological factors. It may also happen that the effort needed to overcome organically based speech diffculties is so great that the patient chooses to be silent rather than to painstakingly stammer a few words. In other words, functionality and organicity are intertwined in some cases.

Chapter 3
The Syndrome of Mutism: Functional Mutism

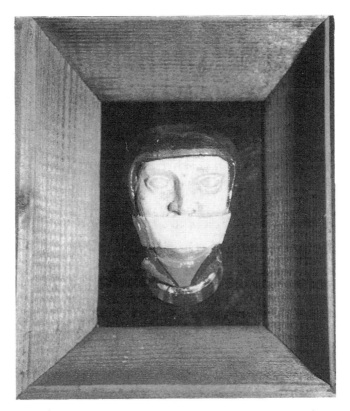

Figure 1. Silence. (From the Senators' Hall in Wawel Castle, Cracow, Poland.)

Selective Mutism

Organicity can be excluded when the patient keeps silent in certain places or in the presence of certain individuals, and uses speech in other places or when interacting with other individuals. This form of functional mutism is usually referred to as 'selective mutism' or 'elective mutism', the two being synonymous.

[Individuals with selective mutism can use speech for communicative purposes, but fail to do so under a number of circumstances where to speak would be the appropriate and expected response.]Because the lack of expressive speech is contingent upon the place the individual is in, or the people he or she is with, some refer to it as 'spatial' or 'situational mutism'.

Selective mutism is a fairly consistent and durable behaviour. It is therefore to be distinguished from the temporary muteness which is often observed in young children when they meet strangers or find themselves in a new environment. For instance, it is not uncommon for a toddler to become silent, and possibly hide behind a parent, when he confronts someone for the first time. Kindergarten children and even those in their first year at school may not say a word during the first few days in school. After they have familiarised themselves with the class situation they start using speech normally again.

Such temporary muteness is not to be confused with selective mutism. The latter does not tend to decrease as the patient becomes better acquainted with the environment. Simple habituation is not enough to make it clear up.

Selective mutism can be observed not only in children but also in adults. Moreover, some children with selective mutism have normal verbal skills, whilst others evidence language delay.

Selective mutism in children with normal command of language

An instance of selective mutism in a boy with normal command of spoken and written language was reported by Strait in 1958. The child, called LeRoy, would use speech with his family but would never speak outside the home. At school he did his silent work carefully but could not be made to answer questions orally, read aloud, recite or take part in choral singing. He used to play alone.

He was referred to a speech therapist, because by school rules he could not advance to the second year until he could read aloud. It took the therapist two sessions to get the boy to show his tongue and teeth.

Gradually, LeRoy could be brought to speak, or read aloud, to a limited number of adults, but he remained completely withdrawn from his contemporaries. Therapy was continued and the child encouraged to associate with other children. At first, he would only use one-word sentences when addressing his playmates. By the end of the second year, his withdrawal and silence were quickly breaking down, and he was socialising more and more. His face became expressive, whereas before he had always shown a blank visage.

Extrafamilial mutism, school mutism and classroom mutism

Typically, the immediate relatives and possibly a few peers are the only people with whom the selectively mute child speaks. Selective mutism is, for the most part, extrafamilial.

Usually, children with extrafamilial mutism are normally talkative at home. However, when strangers are present, they may refrain from speaking even to their parents and siblings.

A few children with extrafamilial mutism prove taciturn at home. These patients use speech sparingly with their close relatives and not at all outside the family circle. Such a case was reported by Bednar (1974). The patient was a 10-year-old boy who 'had never, to anyone's knowledge, spoken a word either in school or outside of his home. The family reported that he spoke very infrequently at home and then primarily to an elder brother'.

There are also selectively mute children who are reported by their parents to be exceedingly loquacious at home. It is not always clear, however, whether this is actually so or whether the parents have a low level of tolerance.

It may happen that one of the parents belongs to the group of people the child never speaks to. For instance, Ruzicka and Sackin (1974) described a 9-year-old girl who would talk to her mother, her brother and a 6-year-old girl who lived in the neighbourhood, but never to her father. Pustrom and Speers' (1964) third patient readily talked to her mother and brother but very little to her father. Scott's (1977) patient did not speak to her grandparents, aunts and uncles, and was very shy of her father, whom she addressed only rarely.

In other cases, the mute behaviour is observed primarily, if not exclusively, in school. For instance, the patient described by Wassing (1973) would talk to his relatives and, as he grew older, also to some strangers, but he remained totally silent in the presence of anyone who had even the slightest connection to his school.

Sometimes, mutism is restricted to classroom situations, as in the case reported by Straughan, Potter and Hamilton (1965).

In rare instances, selective mutism is sex bound. One girl, briefly mentioned by Hayden (1980), stopped talking to men after she had been raped by her mother's boyfriend.

Facial expression and eye contact

Ruzicka and Sackin (1974) report that their patient's face became expressionless whenever she was confronted with someone she would not talk to. The two authors claim that this is typical of selective mutes. Actually, facial voidness was noted in a number of cases, including Strait's (1958). However, lack of facial expression was not observed in the selectively mute twins reported on by Mora, Devault and Schopler (1962); on the contrary, the two girls had 'alert facial expressions'. Also the face of Wassing's (1973) patient was not blank. Rather, the look in the eyes, as well as the body posture, of this boy with absolute school mutism often indicated that he would have liked to associate with his classmates but could not bring himself to join them and speak to them.

A number of selectively mute children have also been reported to have minimal eye contact. They tend to look away when spoken to. For instance, Linda, the mute girl described by Scott (1977), had an expressionless face and she avoided eye contact whenever she was addressed by someone who did not belong to her immediate family. She shunned all kinds of direct communication, whether through speech, gaze or facial expression.

Silent communication

Other selectively mute children do accept silent communication. For instance, Elson *et al.* (1965) observed a young schoolgirl who did her written work exceptionally well but who could not be made to answer orally, to read aloud or to recite in school. Minimal communication with the teacher was possible, however, as the child would shake or nod her head in answer to yes–no questions. Similarly, Hélène, a 7-year-old girl described by Myquel and Granon (1982), did not speak in school but had eye contact with the teacher and used head movements in communication with her. A 14-year-old boy observed by Kupietz and Schwartz (1982) did not speak to his teacher but used gestures when interacting with him, and so did the patient described by Bednar (1974).

It would therefore appear that a number of children with selective mutism avoid verbal as well as non-verbal exchanges with some people. Others, on the contrary, refrain from oral interaction only.

A special use of communicative gestures was observed in the case described by Mora, Devault and Schopler (1962). The two patients were twins. They would use speech between themselves, with their parents and with some peers outside school, but they did not talk to anyone else. Moreover, when someone they normally did not talk to was present, they would resort to a self-made sign language as well as to nods and smiles to communicate with each other. Thus, the patients abstained not only from speaking to a number of people but also from uttering words in the presence of these people.

Reluctant speech

Sometimes, silence is only partial, the child being untalkative rather than mute. Children with partial mutism will respond verbally once in a while or will react briefly to insistent exhortation to speak. However, they may whisper rather than produce voice, or hold a hand before their mouth as they speak. Some authors refer to this type of behaviour as 'reluctant speech'.

Occasionally, reluctant speech is used with one individual whilst others are met with complete silence. For instance, a patient of Shaw's (1971) would from time to time give whispered single-word answers to a particular teacher, when nobody else was present. Otherwise, she remained totally silent outside her home.

A detailed account of reluctant speech associated with other maladaptive behaviours has been given by Wallace (1987). In a Black family with five children, two twin girls first presented with extrafamilial mutism. Eventually they stopped speaking even to their parents and older siblings. They used speech freely between themselves and with their young sister when she came to play in their bedroom, where they spent most of their time.

On rare occasions the twins would answer urgent questions; they would even speak of their own accord when strongly motivated. For instance, they pleaded with their teachers by telephone, when the school staff were considering separating them. Otherwise, they did not talk to people. Indeed, when someone was present they refrained from speaking to each other and communicated by means of glances.

Sex ratio

A number of authors have expressed the view that selective mutism is more frequent in girls than in boys. Others have denied this. Wright et al. (1985) pooled the cases described or mentioned in 47 studies published between 1954 and 1983, and reached a total of 35 males (44%) and 44 females (56%).

To the papers listed by Wright et al. (1985) the articles listed in Table 1 may be added.

Table 1. Sex ratio in selective mutism

Literature	Boys	Girls
Goll (1979)	3	7
Kolvin and Fundudis (1981)	11	13
Morin, Ladouceur and Cloutier (1982)	1	–
Myquel and Granon (1982)	8	6
Schachter (1977)	1	5
Wergeland (1979)	4	7
Wright (1968)	7	17
Wright et al. (1985)	2	1
Youngerman (1979)	1	–
Total	38 (40%)	56 (60%)

Together with the statistics of Wright *et al.* (1985) the statistics presented in the table confirm the view that selective mutism is more frequent in girls than in boys. The reason for the greater incidence among females is not known.

Enuresis and encopresis

Not infrequently children with selective mutism suffer from enuresis. Two of the three patients described by Pustrom and Speers (1964) were still enuretic at the age of 8 years. Three of the six selective mutes reported by Schachter (1977) were enuretic. At the time of examination, they were 4;5, 6;9, and 6;7 years old, respectively. The patient of Hill and Scull (1985) suffered occasionally from enuresis and encopresis until the age of 12 years. Among 11 children with selective mutism Wergeland (1979) found 4 with enuresis and 1 with encopresis. In a group of 24 selectively mute children, Kolvin and Fundudis (1981) found about three times as many bed-wetters and eight times as many soilers as in a control group. Lack of bladder and bowel control was, in fact, the most prominent concomitant of selective mutism in their clinical group.

Do these higher rates of enuresis and encopresis among selective mutes relate to the timidity and apprehensiveness observed in a number of these children? It is well known that fright may prevent the efficient control of the bladder or bowel. Therefore, bashful children may conceivably find it difficult to retain bodily discharges adequately.

Another explanation is forthcoming, however. Speaking, and more specifically answering questions, is a behaviour that has to be learned and practised by the child in order to facilitate social integration. The same holds true of bladder and bowel control. In company, speaking and toileting are required demeanours. Mute children not infrequently fail to fully master these two psychophysiological behaviours. For instance, Anna, the mute girl described by Goll (1979), did not speak a word on her first day in kindergarten and did not partake in any of the classroom activities. However, at some point she stood up and urinated in the classroom. The mute girl described by Chethik (1977) had not yet achieved complete control of her bodily discharges at 6;5 years of age. At the beginning of her first therapy session 'she wetted herself and the chair'.

Mutism and enuresis–encopresis may possibly be indicative of lack of social adjustment. They may point to a failure to comply with the group's norms and to answer its expectations, or else they may proceed from an unconscious reluctance to grow up, to cease to be an infant. In this condition it may be significant that some selectively mute children, whilst no longer incontinent, still require adult assistance, whereas their peers already manage for themselves. For instance, at 6 years of age, a boy described by Wassing (1973) still needed his mother's help for his stools, and a 7-year-old boy mentioned by Goll (1979) insisted on being held like a baby when using the toilet.

Psychoanalysts consider that in the child who is toilet-trained speech provides an avenue of 'outerance' to replace the free urination and defaecation of babyhood. As Sharpe (1940) put it: 'The activity of speaking is substituted for the physical activity now restricted at other openings of the body.' Accordingly, if speech is inhibited, sphincter control becomes difficult.

These various explanations of the greater occurrence of enuresis–encopresis among selective mutes are not mutually exclusive. A child may exhibit insufficient bladder and bowel control for several reasons, and different patients may be enuretic or encopresic for different reasons.

The dynamics of selective mutism

Analysis of the numerous cases of selective mutism reported in the literature shows that selectively mute children are not all alike.

Some of the children appear shy and restricted outside the family circle or at home when strangers are present. They seem to be using their mutism to keep others at a distance, to reduce the demands of the environment, and to escape competition. Apparently they feel that by keeping their own counsel they can become unnoticeable and hide from the outside world. In a way they resemble the small animals which freeze in the presence of danger. In addition, some of them may refrain from talking to strangers in an effort to ignore their existence and thus to render them inoffensive.

These children tend to react with tears or complete withdrawal if anyone seeks to coerce them to speak. When pressured to talk, Hill and Scull's (1985) patient would develop tremors in his head and hands and become inaccessible.

At home, probably because they feel more at ease and have better control of the situation, the children may exhibit a totally different behaviour. Not only do they use speech but they may be demanding or wild. Indeed, some of them can be really tyrannical.

A number of selective mutes appear overly attached to their mother. They feel lost, insecure and unhappy when separated from her. Their mutism seems to be an attempt to control somewhat a frightening environment. Their silence appears to be primarily an anxiety-reducing strategy.

Selective mutism may also be an expression of the child's objection to being separated from his or her mother, a kind of silent protest against being sent to school. A case in point was reported by Pustrum and Speers in 1964. At 3 years of age, the young patient had manifested intense separation fear when put in the Sunday school nursery while his mother attended the regular services. He would kick, scream and call for his mother. When she did not appear, he would become quiet and sullen, and would withdraw from the other children. This behaviour was repeated when he entered kindgarten at the age of 5 years. Separation difficulties occurred again 1 year later as he began state school. From the first day on he refused to talk to anyone. At home, on the other hand, he was loquacious and tyrannical.

Not infrequently, selective mutism seems to be both a fear-reducing reaction and a protest against being left in a situation that cannot be coped with.

In some instances, the mutism appears to be part of the child's negativism. The young patient is not only mute but also oppositional. His silence is an expression of hostility. At the same time it may be an attention-gaining device.

It may also be a means to achieve power. Gwen, an 8-year-old girl described by Pustrom and Speers (1964), talked readily to her mother and brother but very little to her father. He tended to comply with all her whims in the hope that she would talk more frequently to him.

In the case of twins, silence may offer the advantage that it increases the children's feeling of forming a close unit separated from those around them. In their report on selective mutism in identical twins, Mora, Devault and Schopler (1962) noted that the 'symptom seemed to represent a kind of magic, symbolic tie between them'.

It appears, then, that the personality structure of selectively mute children is not uniform. Moreover, the dynamics of selective mutism may be different in different patients.

Parental attitude

Some parents of selectively mute children appear unconcerned about the problem and not anxious to have it treated. For instance, the mother of the twins described by Mora, Devault and Schopler (1962) and the mother of the girl observed by Elson *et al.* (1965) sought help only at the school's insistent request.

In fact, many cases of extrafamilial mutism do not come into evidence until the child starts to go to school. For instance, in the epidemiological study carried out by Kolvin and Fundudis (1981), the average age when the electively mute children were first diagnosed was 6;10 years (with a standard deviation of 1,3 years).

As long as the child spends most of the time with his family, his lack of oral expression in the presence of strangers is often considered by the parents to be of little consequence. It is dismissed as a form of shyness, which, it is assumed, the child will eventually outgrow. This unconcern on the part of the parents does not favour the elimination of the mute behaviour.

Indeed, at times, the child's mutism is actually reinforced by a parent, who may himself have been a mute for some time or may consider silence an appropriate reaction to life's vexations. For instance, the father of Johnny, an electively mute boy described by Pustrom and Speers (1964), recalled that as a child he spoke infrequently. The mother of the twins observed by Mora, Devault and Schopler (1962) 'often did not feel like talking if an unpleasant subject was brought up', and she tended to admire her daughters for keeping silent outside the house. When she was angry at her husband, the mother of Kaplan and Escoll's (1973) first patient would refuse to talk to him for weeks at a time. The mother of Goll's (1979) third patient had not only shown selective mutism as a child, but as a married woman hardly ever talked to her husband and did not feel that it was a great disadvantage for her daughter not to speak outside the home.

The father of one of Pustrom and Speer's (1964) patients 'had an intense fear of speaking in public because of embarrassment over what he might say, or questions that might be asked which he would be unable to answer. He thus avoided discussions, and rarely volunteered an opinion outside the immediate family circle'. As for the father of the selectively mute twins described by Kroppenberg (1987), he found that his daughter's muteness protected them against the buffets of life.

When the mother is of the possessive type, she may be inclined to favour her child's extrafamilial mutism, because it tends to isolate him from the outside world and to render him less susceptible to the influence of others.

In some cases, extreme bashfulness and difficulty in communicating orally is a familial trait. For instance, the maternal grandmother and the mother of Linda, a selectively mute girl described by Scott (1977), had both been extremely shy in childhood. Linda's eldest brother had separation difficulties when first admitted to school, and Linda's other two siblings did not begin speaking to their teachers until their second year at school.

Sometimes, the relatives of the mute child need some warming-up before they can start talking to someone they do not know very well. Youngerman (1979) reports that when he began meeting with his mute patient's family at their house, they would sit for 10–15 minutes 'in utter and seemingly unembarrassed silence'. Then spontaneous activity was resumed and talking gradually evolved, except from the mother who remained taciturn.

Such observations have led some researchers to assume the possibility of a genetic disposition to mutism. It could be, however, that mutism here is not so much a matter of inheritance as a matter of imitation.

Selective mutism as a family problem

A number of clinicians are of the opinion that selective mutism in children is, in fact, a family problem. The family structure, the role distribution within it and the example set by the parents contribute to the occurrence and maintenance of the silent behaviour. In Pustrom and Speer's (1964) view 'elective mutism in the child (is) the symptom expression of the family conflict'.

However, a number of clinical reports show that the familial constellation is not always disturbed, and matrimonial discord not invariably present. For instance, in a group of 21 families with a selectively mute child, Wright (1968) found 5 which were basically normal. In 10 out of 23 families, Kolvin and Fundudis (1981) observed no major personality or psychiatric problem and no marital dysharmony.

Even though they do not live in a disturbed family, some children with extrafamilial mutism may fail to find at home the warmth, comfort and reassurance which they need to verbally confront the outer world.

In some cases, then, the child's selective mutism appears related to, and may in fact be the reflection of, tensions within the family. In other cases, the child may be missing the familial back-up which he needs to deal with the outside world. In still other cases, it looks as if the child's own personality structure is the main causal factor.

Familial secret

In a number of cases, extrafamilial mutism may be reinforced by the existence of a secret within the family, of something one should be careful not to talk about to strangers. In the second case reported by Myquel and Granon (1982), the patient's mother did not want anyone to know that her daughter was not her biological child, but an adopted child. In the first case reported by Pustrom and Speers (1964), a paternal grandmother had psychiatric treatment and the young patient was constantly reminded to tell her nothing about the family for fear that she in turn might tell her psychiatrist. In Pustrom and Speers's second case, the patient's mother was terribly afraid that her son might one day discover, and later divulge, that her own mother had had an illegitimate child. She was also apprehensive that her child (who, it should be remembered, had extrafamilial mutism!) might tell others about intimacies between her and her husband. In Pustrom and Speers's third case, the patient's mother was concerned that her husband or children 'might say the wrong thing'.

Reporting on a school with an unusually high proportion of selectively mute children, Lesser-Katz (1986) also underscored the existence of familial secrets. The pupils came mostly from poor families who depended on state assistance. The fact that the father earned some money doing odd jobs could not be divulged. Violence within the family was frequent and this, too, had to be kept private.

It is therefore conceivable that, in a number of cases, the child's tendency to taciturnity is enhanced by constant reminders to keep something secret.

Familial isolation

Another factor which, in some instances of extrafamilial mutism, seems to play a role in the occurrence of the disorder is the relative isolation of the family. At times, this isolation is purely geographical, the family living in some remote area or in an isolated house, as a consequence of which the young patient has but limited contacts with the outside world before being sent to school. He is unaccustomed to seeing strangers and to associating with people other than his immediate relatives. Going to school may therefore amount to entering a strange, unknown and threatening world to which the frightened child reacts with withdrawal and silence, retiring into his protective shell, as a snail would do.

The isolation may also be social, as is the case with a number of immigrant families, who do not completely master the language of their new homeland and find it difficult (or are reluctant) to adjust to their new environment. The negative attitude of his parents towards the outside world may conceivably play a part in the occurrence of a child's extrafamilial mutism, especially if he finds himself language handicapped outside the home. It is therefore not surprising that Bradley and Sloman (1975) should have found a greater proportion of electively mute children in immigrant, non-English speaking families than in English-speaking families of the Toronto area.

A striking instance of extrafamilial mutism in which failure to adapt to the new social and linguistic environment played an important role, was reported by Shaw (1971). The patient was an 11-year-old girl whose Dutch family had moved to an English-speaking community in Canada when she was a toddler. Unlike her sister and brothers, she did not begin to speak English. She used Dutch exclusively and continued to do so even after English had become the language generally spoken in her home. She did not talk to anyone outside her family circle although on written testing her proficiency in English proved to be age appropriate.

Goll (1979) contended that all selectively mute children come from what he called 'ghetto families', i.e. families who in one way or another are segregated from the community or occupy a marginal position in society. This is probably a gross exaggeration. Not all selectively mute children have on examination been found to live in an ill-integrated, outcast or otherwise isolated family. But some of them undoutedly have. For instance, in a group of 11 children with selective mutism Wergeland (1979) noted that 8 came from families who 'lived in social aloofness in remote homes'.

Although the geographical or social isolation of the family may conceivably be a facilitative factor in the occurrence of selective mutism, its importance should not be exaggerated. The Gibbon family described by Wallace (1987) had few social contacts. Yet, only two of the five children presented with mutism. Probably familial isolation plays a role only in the presence of other factors. In the case of June and Jennifer Gibbon, for instance, it seems to have only added to the pathological interdependence of the twin sisters.

Reactions of the environment

Whilst the immediate relatives may be surprisingly tolerant of, or unconcerned about, the child's selective mutism, other people generally resent it. The child's silence is often regarded as a form of stubbornness or hostility, and is negatively reacted to. It is considered deliberate and a cause for punishment. Indeed, the irritation it provokes may lead to the application of stringent measures to break it.

Even therapists may find it difficult to cope with the child's lack of speech. As the report by Mora, Devault and Schopler (1962) indicates, they may feel frustrated by the patient's persisting silence. Ruzicka (in Ruzicka and Sackin, 1974) confesses that she felt thwarted by her client's unresponsiveness. She had great difficulty in enduring this chronic assault upon her ego. Youngerman (1979) also pointed out the countertransference which the patient's mutism may engender in the therapist. Maybe this reaction is not unlike the narcissistic wound which we usually feel when the person to whom we have put a question fails to give any sort of answer, or when our speech partner fails to signal from time to time that he keeps listening to our report.

On the other hand, once the environment has become accustomed to the patient's silence and has accepted it, this very tolerance may in itself contribute to the maintenance of mutism. The child is expected to keep silent, so why should he startle everybody by beginning to speak? Especially if his classmates readily act as his spokesmen and the teacher is willing to accept written answers or head nods instead of oral responses. A number of researchers, and notably Straughan (1968), have laid stress on this reinforcement by the environment of the child's long-standing mutism.

Therapy

Essentially two types of therapeutic approaches have been used with selectively mute children. The first type focuses on the symptom – mutism – and tries to eliminate it gradually. The other type focuses on the mechanism which is supposed to underlie the absence of expressive speech.

Therapies concentrating on the symptom are for the most part behaviour modification techniques. Three different operant conditioning strategies have been employed. In one approach, the clinician first attempts to establish direct verbal contact with the child in a one-to-one situation. Once the contact is established, he lets in a third person unobtrusively. After a while, he tries to have the child talk (or read out) to the third person. When this is achieved, other interlocutors are gradually phased in. At times, as in cases reported by Goll (1979), hypnosis is used initially to establish verbal contact between the patient and the therapist.

An application of this technique (not involving hypnosis) has been reported by Rosenbaum and Kellman (1973). The patient was a third-year pupil who did not speak in school. First, speech with the speech therapist in a one-to-one setting was established. A simple shaping procedure was used to this end. The subject began by responding to questions with head noddings. Following this, she was required to make some verbal sound to receive her reward, which consisted of sweets and social approval. Gradually she was required to produce words and then longer and longer sentences. At the end of this phase, the sweet reward was discontinued and only social reinforcement given.

After approximately eight sessions with the speech therapist, when conversation was occurring easily, the subject was persuaded to read aloud from her reading book. The oral reading was tape-recorded and the subject required to take the recording to her classroom and to play it back to her teacher and classmates. During playback, the girl spontaneously followed in her reader, silently mouthing the words.

After this had been done three times, the teacher made a visit to the therapy room while the patient was conversing with her therapist. The teacher asked a number of questions, which the girl answered orally. The teacher then walked the child to the classroom. The two of them conversed all the way. Later that week, the teacher went to the girl's home for lunch and spoke with her there.

In subsequent therapy sessions, more and more classmates were let in and read aloud with the patient. The reading group thus formed could soon be transferred to the regular classroom, where the subject not only read aloud in unison with her fellow students but also asked the teacher a few questions.

The patient then started to invite classmates to the therapy sessions to play guessing games with her and the therapist. This procedure continued for about 10 weeks until all the children in the class had had an opportunity to participate in the speechroom sessions. During this time, the teacher was structuring small group situations which included the patient and required her to speak in the classroom. She consistently praised the girl's verbal behaviour with words and close physical contact. By the end of this phase, the patient would answer questions directly put to her in front of the entire class. Treatment was terminated at this point.

Follow-up some 2.5 months later found that the girl had remained normally verbal at school. Indeed, in small groups she tended to dominate the conversation.

In a slightly different approach, the mother is initially involved. She is requested to have the child talk to her outside the home, for instance in a vacant classroom. After a few sessions, the clinician unobtrusively enters the room and gradually increases his proximity to the patient. Then he asks the patient questions by way of his mother.

The next step is to have the child answer the questions which the clinician puts directly to him. The presence of the mother is progressively reduced. When the child speaks freely to the clinician, more and more outsiders are let in and the child is encouraged to speak to them also.

This therapy is sometimes called 'stimulus-fading programme'. An application of it has been reported by Kupietz and Schwartz (1982):

> The stimulus-fading program was begun with the mother engaging the boy in his favorite card games in a vacant classroom. In the fifth session, a teacher with whom the boy was familiar was introduced into the program. Initially she sat in a corner of the room out of the boy's view pretending to be preoccupied with her own work. Gradually she moved her seat closer to the table where the boy and his mother conversed. By the tenth session she was seated alongside the table; the boy stopped talking and refused to play the game. By the fourteenth session, he seemed more relaxed and began to whisper to his mother in the teacher's presence.
>
> In subsequent sessions, he resumed normal conversation with his mother and had begun to respond to questions posed by the teacher and relayed by his mother. Direct verbal responses to the teacher were achieved by session 21. The mother was completely 'faded out' of the program over the next 10 sessions. By this time, the boy responded readily to his teacher. In all, the stimulus-fading program required approximately 31 sessions distributed over a three-month period.

In a case reported by Reid *et al.* (1967), the stimulus-fading programme was applied in one day with a girl suffering from extrafamilial mutism. By the end of the day, the patient would answer questions from various members of the speech clinic. A week later, the mother reported that her daughter had begun to talk to people outside the family, such as her Sunday school teacher and friends of her parents.

Therapeutic success is not always achieved so easily. Transfer of the speech behaviour from the therapy room to the classroom may prove particularly difficult. For instance, in a case reported by Colligan, Colligan and Dillard (1977), a structured procedure directly involving the classmates had to be designed in order to have the speechroom verbal behaviour generalise to the classroom situation. The authors concluded that the instigating and reinforcing behaviour of peers may be an important variable in the treatment of classroom mutism.

In the third approach, the therapy takes place directly in the classroom with the teacher as agent of change. Initially, the mute pupil is exhorted to give minimal non-verbal responses (such as hand raising or head nodding). Then a minimal verbal behaviour is required of him and rewarded by the teacher whenever it occurs. Demands are gradually stepped up until normal or near normal verbal behaviour in the classroom is obtained. In individual cases, the first stage, that of minimal non-verbal responses, may be dropped.

Halpern, Hammond and Cohen (1971), who favoured this third approach, outlined their programme as follows:

> Preliminary conferences are convened for a discussion of the child, of the dynamics of his functional mutism, of the tactics to be used for getting the child to speak, and of the contingencies for which the teacher must be prepared. As soon as a plan is agreed on, the child is readied by his teacher with a statement of expectations and consequences the day before the procedures go into effect. This information is imparted in the presence of his classmates so that they are aware of the planned nature of the confrontation. Initially, what the child is asked to do is to speak a preselected word in order to be released from the classroom by this teacher. As long as he remains mute, both he and the teacher, who is most familiar with the child, remain in the room after the child's classmates have departed. The teacher busies herself with some work and, from time to time, reminds the child that he can go out on cue. As quickly as the desired for word is spoken, he is praised for his courage and is sent on his way. Subsequently, he must, at the very least, offer the chosen word whenever he wishes to leave the room. In time, the teacher gradually steps up demands for verbal participation in the classroom until a more or less normal performance is achieved.

According to Straughan, Potter and Hamilton (1965), who fruitfully used this technique with a 14-year-old boy, an operant rate greater than zero is prerequisite, i.e. that the child should not be totally unresponsive in the classroom before treatment begins. As a matter of fact, the method was used successfully by Bauermeister and Jemail (1975) and by Morin, Ladouceur and Cloutier (1982) in two cases of reluctant speech at school.

Generally clinicians who use behaviour modification procedures with selectively mute children resort to tangible and social rewards to reinforce the desired behaviour. In a case reported by Shaw (1971), however, an aversive stimulus was used. In an early attempt to cure the patient's extrafamilial mutism, injections of amobarbital sodium and of methamphetamine hydrochloride had been given. These injections had had little effect on the patient's verbal behaviour but it had been discovered that she intensely disliked them. A graded programme of desensitisation was instituted which used the injections as a conditioned aversive stimulus. Whenever the girl failed to meet the day's minimal speech requirement, she was given an injection. The patient's dislike of shots, later associated with positive social reinforcement, enabled her to complete the therapy programme and to achieve a normal speech behaviour.

In general, behaviour modification therapies for selective mutism are carefully graded and proceed slowly, one step at a time. Not infrequently they have to be extended over a fairly long period of time, and progress may be slow. For instance, the patient may at some time start to react verbally but may do so in a barely audible whisper, and quite some time may elapse before the therapist succeeds in turning this whisper into loud speech. Speedy elimination of selective mutism, as in the case reported by Reid *et al.* (1967), is exceptional (see p. 28).

Whilst some clinicians advocate behaviour modification therapies in the treatment of selective mutism, others favour psychotherapy. In the case of the twins described by Mora, Devault and Schopler (1962) and in the three cases reported by Pustrom and Speers (1964), this approach proved beneficial. In Smayling's case E (1959), it failed to improve the patient's verbal behaviour, although it was extended for 3 years.

In the case described by Mora, Devault and Schopler (1962) the twins were encouraged to accept their own individuality and to be independent of one another as well as of their mother. The mother was exhorted to forsake her control of the twins through their symptom and to let them develop their social activities individually.

In the cases reported by Pustrom and Speers (1964), the focus with the patient was on his potentially aggressive impulses and their anticipated consequences as well as on his need to maintain a dependency relationship with his mother. The focus with the parent was on the marital discord and on the mother's need to maintain an unusually strong bond with her child. In addition, the conflict over talking and its consequences was thoroughly aired.

As psychotherapy progressed, the patients of Mora, Devault and Schopler and of Pustrum and Speers started to talk to an ever increasing number of people but remained silent in the presence of their therapist, with whom they continued to communicate in writing. This may have been a consequence of the permissiveness of the therapist, who did not insist on obtaining speech during therapy sessions. Indeed, in the Pustrom and Speers cases, the therapist's general attitude was: 'I can help you whether you talk or not.'

Wergeland (1979) reported on four selective mutes who received individual psychotherapy as in-patients for a period of 8 months, 2 years (two children) and 3 years, respectively. One of these children was discharged unimproved after 2 years of therapy; the other three were symptom free at the end of treatment. Two further children received psychotherapy as out-patients. They were not improved after 3.5 and 4 years respectively of treatment.

Follow-up examination, 8–16 years later, indicated that all six patients were now symptom free. The three patients who had benefited from therapy had had no relapse.

The other three patients had become more verbal in connection with a change in environment. They could conquer their mutism after they started a new life with people they had never met before. This seems to confirm the view that when selective mutism has been present for quite some time, it may be difficult for the patient to relinquish a behaviour which has become an integral part of his daily life and to which his entourage is now fully accustomed. People who retreat into mutism may one day find themselves trapped in it.

Some selectively mute teenagers seem to remain mute mainly because they view themselves, and are viewed by others, as mutes. Ruth, one of the two twin girls described by Mora, Devault and Schopler (1962), indicated after therapy had started to have some positive effect, that she now felt comfortable in talking to people who did not know her at all, whereas she still found it difficult to talk to people to whom she had failed to respond verbally in the past. On another occasion, her sister, when asked why she did not talk in school, had written: 'When I was small, I just did not want to talk for some reason I don't know. Now I am older, I still don't know. I am afraid what people will say if I start now.'

Similarly, after he had been treated for some time, Bednar's (1974) patient began to attend an after-school tutoring programme. He had never met the tutor and supervisors of this programme before and had no difficulty in talking to them. But he still could not talk to his regular teacher and regular classmates. He felt that they would be angry with him if he now started to speak to them.

One of Wergeland's (1979) patients must have felt the same. Despite 2 years of psychotherapy as an in-patient this girl remained mute. She managed to complete secondary school and domestic science college without speaking. Then she stayed with her mother, helping her in the house. She spoke to her but kept silent outside the house. Eventually, she took a job in a town where she had no acquaintances, and started to exhibit a normal verbal behaviour. However, she continued to be silent in her home-town when she returned for weekend visits.

It appears, then, that even after they have managed, spontaneously or under the influence of therapy, to establish a normal pattern of verbal behaviour, patients may still refrain from talking to people who have always known them as mutes.

Moreover, elimination of selective mutism is no guarantee that social behaviour will be totally adequate. Although they had all stopped being mute, only two of Wergeland's six patients appeared on follow-up examination to be well adjusted. One had moderate difficulties in the form of contact problems and a tendency to isolation, two were neurotic, and one was psychotic.

Somewhat better outcome was reported by Reed (1963). His four patients received psychotherapy for elective mutism and became more verbal. Later, they all adjusted reasonably well to life, but continued to show minor psychogenic abnormalities and a lack of social drive.

When the literature on the treatment of selective mutism is surveyed, the impression obtained is that behaviour modification techniques have achieved a somewhat greater rate of success than psychodynamic procedures, For instance, Scott (1977) reported on a 5-year-old selectively mute girl whose verbal behaviour could not be changed through psychotherapy but could be improved through operant procedures.

It could, however, be that failures to eliminate selective mutism by means of behaviour modification therapy are just as frequent as failures to eliminate it by means of psychotherapy, but are less often reported in the literature. Moreover, success with desensitisation may be more apparent than real, as there can be symptom substitution: mutism disappears but is replaced by another deviant behaviour. Halpern, Hammond and Cohen (1971) have warned against this danger and recommended that programmes of behaviour modification should be carried out with due attention paid to the child's limited adaptive powers. Specifically, if the patient uses silence as an avoidance strategy to decrease his fears, the therapist should make him sense that speech can be used as a valid anxiety-reducing alternative.

Accordingly, it does not seem possible to decide which of the two approaches – behavioural, symptom-oriented therapy *vs* cause-oriented psychotherapy – is the more efficient with selectively mute children.

Sometimes the two methods are combined, as in the case reported by Wassing (1973). The patient was a 12-year-old boy called John, who had total school mutism. Behaviour modification therapy was used to instigate speech with the therapist, and psychotherapy, supplemented by behaviour modification therapy, to obtain generalisation of speech to school situations.

It took no less than 83 sessions to have the patient converse with his therapist. The first step was to have the boy read from a book into a microphone connected to a tape-recorder. The patient was left alone while recording himself. The therapist would enter the room after the patient had made the recording, and he would listen to it together with the patient.

During the first few sessions, John only whispered into the microphone. It took eight sessions before he could phonate.

Once loud reading had been consolidated, the patient was required to make the recording while the therapist sat in a corner of the room reading a book. The presence of the therapist caused the patient to regress to whispering. Twenty-four sessions were necessary before reading could be done again in a loud voice. Then the therapist changed his position in the room. He sat closer and closer to the patient and started to look at him during recording.

When John could read aloud with the therapist sitting in front of him and looking at him, he was asked a few questions. He would write down his answers and then read aloud what he had written. It took eight sessions before he could read aloud his answers with normal vocal volume.

Next, the patient was requested to answer yes–no questions directly, while continuing to write down and read out longer answers. Eighteen sessions were necessary before this could be effected easily.

At the next stage, the boy had to read aloud each answer and then to repeat it without looking at the written text. Finally, he could be induced to answer the therapist's questions directly. In all, this behaviour therapy took a whole year.

Once John was able to answer his therapist's questions, psychotherapy was introduced. While still supporting and socially rewarding the patient's effort to speak, the therapist started to discuss his reasons for keeping silent in school. As psychotherapy proceeded, the boy began to speak to a limited number of people in school provided he could meet them individually.

In order to have John speak in the classroom, a new desensitisation procedure had to be applied. At first, the boy was required to prepare a short lecture on a topic he liked and to tape-record it in his usual therapy room at the hospital. The recording was played back to the class, at first in the patient's absence, later while he was present.

Next, the boy was induced to read aloud from a book and to record himself in the empty classroom. The recording was played back to the entire class in his presence.

At the next stage, the patient recorded himself in the presence of one classmate. Then more and more pupils were admitted to the classroom while John was recording himself. Next, the patient and four classmates tape-recorded a play with five characters in it. Then John could be induced to play a word game with his four partners. After the game had been repeated with other pupils, the boy proved able to read aloud and to answer questions orally in the classroom.

Verbal behaviour finally normalised after the patient had been persuaded to play the announcer in a show put up at the hospital. By the time this was achieved, John had been in therapy for 3.5 years.

Rosenberg and Lindblad (1978) have contended that behavioural therapy is ineffective with selectively mute children if the patient's parents are not given psychotherapy, or at least psychological counselling, at the same time. Clinical facts do not entirely bear out this statement. In a number of cases, including the one reported by Straughan, Potter and Hamilton (1965), improvement of the patient's verbal behaviour could be achieved without involving the parents or giving them therapy. But obviously, when it is felt that the parents' attitude or behaviour tends to reinforce the child's mutism, it is necessary to change the family's functioning if the child is to make any progress at all.

Spontaneous recovery

A number of selectively mute children eventually outgrow their mutism. However, as a case reported by Wergeland (1979) shows, this may not be until the patient is an adult and spends some of his time in new environments. Accordingly, the adoption of a wait-and-see position in the presence of a child with selective mutism does not seem justified. If nothing is done about it, the child is likely to grow out of it. But this may take time, and meanwhile mutism will slow down the child's academic progress and hamper his social integration. On the other hand, early intervention, preferably in kindergarten, is often successful without being too difficult, as a study by Wright *et al.* (1985) shows. It appears desirable, therefore, to identify selectively mute children as early as possible and to refer them without delay to an experienced clinician for assessment and therapy.

Selective mutism in children with language delay

In the cases of selective mutism discussed above, the young patients had age-appropriate language command. There are, however, also children with selective mutism who have defective speech. When talking to their relatives or to people with whom they feel at ease, they evidence speech or language delay. In a group of 24 selectively mute children, Kolvin and Fundudis (1981) found 12 whose command of language was below norm.

Selective mutes with underdeveloped verbal skills are often reported to have been late in starting to speak.

Selective mutism in children with language delay may result primarily from an unconscious desire to avoid a narcissistic wound. Due to their limited abilities these children may be afraid of speaking to strangers who might ridicule them or become angry at their lack of verbal agility. At home, they feel more at ease because their language delay is accepted.

In a number of cases, improvement can be brought about by gaining the child's confidence and then involving him in an intensive individual speech therapy programme. As the child sees his verbal skills develop, he becomes more self-assured and progressively starts using speech outside the home situation. Such a case was reported by Launay and Soulé (1952). The patient was a 6-year-old girl whose command of expressive speech was very limited. At home, she used the little speech she had, together with gestures. Outside the home, she never spoke. After 2 years of therapy, her speech was considerably better. Nevertheless, she remained rather taciturn at school.

At times, however, as in case D reported by Smayling (1959), therapy unexpectedly renders the child garrulous. It is as if the young patient now feels elated and wants to revel in the newly acquired language skills.

Children with selective mutism and language delay, whilst not very verbal, may nevertheless be vocal. Myquel and Granon (1982) reported the case of a toddler who had extrafamilial mutism together with underdeveloped language skills but who liked to imitate non-verbal noises. Although he did not talk to strangers, he occasionally attempted to communicate with them by using pitch variations.

In addition to language delay, a number of selectively mute children have some degree of mental handicap. For instance, the mixed verbal IQs (Terman–Merrill revision of the Binet) of the four mutes described by Reed (1963) were 72, 60, 61 and 70 respectively, whilst their non-verbal IQs (Alexander Performance Scale) were 70, 88, 60 and 95. Two of the three patients reported by Kupietz and Schwartz (1982) also showed moderate handicap. The selectively mute boy described by Straughan, Potter and Hamilton (1965) was in a school for the mentally handicapped. His IQ as measured by the Leiter International Performance Scale was 52. Several earlier tests with the WISC (Wechsler Intelligence Scale for Children) and Stanford–Binet had indicated IQs from 60 to 65.

In a group of 21 selectively mute children, Kolvin and Fundudis (1981) found 4 (19%) with a performance IQ lower than 70. Reed (1963) hypothesised that in cases with mental handicap extrafamilial mutism may be reinforced by the child's wish to conceal his intellectual limitations. Conversely, by restricting the child's participation in classroom activities, mutism may conceivably decrease the child's academic achievement. In this connection, it is of interest that the schoolwork of both the patient of Straughan, Potter and Hamilton (1965) and the patient of Bauermeister and Jemail (1975) improved as their classroom mutism receded.

In Hill and Scull's (1985) case, selective mutism was accompanied by hypoactivity at school. The patient failed to fulfil a number of tasks schoolchildren are normally expected to carry out. As a consequence, after 3 years in elementary (primary) school he was still performing at a preschool level. As his selective mutism receded under the influence of therapy, his non-verbal activities tended to normalise and his social skills to improve.

Late onset of speech without actual language delay

At times, electively mute children are encountered who started to speak late but with an age-appropriate command of language and speech. It is as if the child at first could not bring himself to address even his close relatives verbally. He eventually opened up enough to speak to an intimate circle of people but to nobody else. Such a case was reported by Wassing (1973). His patient did not speak until he was 2 years old, but shortly after he started to speak he could be readily understood. However, he talked only to members of his family. He never spoke to other people.

Selective mutism in adults

Selective mutism may be observed not only in children but also in adults. In adults, however, selective mutism nearly always manifests itself in relation to one specific individual or to a very small group of individuals, not in relation to an environment. Moreover, mutism is generally clearly deliberate. For instance, after some disagreement or quarrel, a person may decide no longer to talk to another person. The two people then cease to be 'on speaking terms'.

Such a situation may prevail between people who are not closely associated, as between neighbours, and therefore be of little consequence. In other cases, mutism characterises the reciprocal behaviour of two persons living together.

There exist two famous literary illustrations of this situation. One is by the Belgian writer Georges Simenon. In the novel entitled *Le Chat* (*The Cat*) Simenon described two elderly people, Emile and Marguerite, who marry one another to escape solitude. They do not really love each other.

During the first night together, Emile attempts to have sexual intercourse with his wife, but she remains unresponsive and he gives up, never to try again.

In fact, the partners do not get along very well with one another. For instance, Emile has a cat, of which he is very fond, but Marguerite cannot stand her husband's pet, and one day she poisons it. This infuriates Emile who kills his wife's parrot. Emile's reaction upsets Marguerite. In writing she informs her husband that she will not talk to him any more and does not want him to talk to her.

Till Marguerite's death a few years later, the spouses continue to live together but without ever speaking to one another. However, from time to time they exchange short written messages.

A similar situation was depicted by A.J. Cronin in the novel entitled *The Adventures of a Black Bag*. Two unmarried sisters live together in the ancestral house. One day they quarrel about a trifle. Neither of them will yield and they stop talking to one another. During the ensuing 15 years they never speak to each other. When they need to communicate they resort to written language.

Interestingly, in both instances only oral communication is suppressed. Despite their animosity, the partners are willing to exchange written messages. This suggests that written language is considered by some people to be a more neutral and more impersonal means of communication than spoken language. The latter presupposes a partner, who is physically present, and to whom the speaker directly relates through the very fact that he is speaking to him.

Written language, on the contrary, does not imply the physical presence of a partner. Indeed, it is typically the language of absence. Therefore, it does not create the same close relationship between two people as spoken language. Accordingly, it can still be used by individuals who no longer want to have intimacy with one another.

The dissociation between oral and written communication could be clearly felt in a case of selective mutism reported by Tolentino (1957). This psychiatrist had under his care an intelligent young woman who a few years earlier had gone through an acute psychotic spell. Ever since, she had been withdrawn and not very active, and had had few affective bonds. She would use spoken language with friends and relatives, but would keep absolutely silent during psychiatric sessions. However, she was willing to answer her psychiatrist's questions in writing.

Using written language, she explained that she tended to be untalkative. Indeed, at times she would remain completely mute. Silence expressed her passive revolt against her environment. She felt that speech would bind her to her interlocutor and she wanted to avoid all bonds, all close relationships. She could converse in writing because, she said, writing did not commit her to a partner. In her view, writing was like talking to oneself. It did not imply responsibilities towards someone else.

Speaking, on the contrary, was hazardous. The words uttered could kill the interlocutor. At the same time, the speaker exposed himself to the reactions of his listener.

Tolentino's patient seemed further to feel that the opening of her mouth might enable others to penetrate into her body, to reach her private secret self. She appeared to shudder at the mere thought of such a violation.

Obviously, very ancient fears and taboos were at work here. To begin with, what comes out of someone's body has from time immemorial been considered potentially harmful and therefore to be feared. The air on which someone speaks may hurt others, because it comes out of the speaker's body. For the same reason, the words he utters may injure his partner.

Concurrently, the breath coming out of somebody's mouth represents this person's individuality. This is why the Latin word 'anima' meant not only 'breath', but also 'being' and 'soul'. Therefore, when he opens his mouth or when he speaks, an individual tends to lay himself bare. In a way, he delivers himself over to his partner. This is probably why during the first therapy session a 3-year-old boy with extrafamilial mutism and language delay, described by Myquel and Granon (1982), held his breath until he turned blue and nearly fainted.

Also, when someone opens his mouth, he provides an entrance to his body and hence to his inner self. The mouth is the doorway to the inmost being. This may be the reason why a deep kiss involving the introduction of the tongue tip into the partner's mouth is called a 'soul kiss'.

Exposing oneself by opening one's mouth can be risky. Others might penetrate you, and this intrusion might destroy your integrity and ruin your self-defence. This is probably why LeRoy, the schoolboy with selective mutism described by Strait (1958), during the first two therapy sessions stubbornly refused to let the therapist see his teeth and tongue. Similarly, the 18-year-old patient briefly described by Critchley (1970, p. 386), when seen for the first time at the hospital, could not be persuaded to open his mouth, to whistle, to blow out a lighted match, or to accept and eat a biscuit. Also a little girl with extrafamilial mutism, when first sent to kindergarten, wept continuously but with closed mouth (Schachter, 1977). As for the selectively mute boy whom Goll (1979) took into his house, he used to keep his jaws so firmly clenched that his masseters had become very prominent. In the case reported by Shaw (1971), it was not until treatment had begun to be effective and mutism had started to decrease that dental work could be performed. Previously, the patient had stubbornly refused to open her mouth.

When, in the early stages of therapy, Bednar's (1974) young patient was requested to make a sound to accompany each written answer he gave, he at first produced clicks with his mouth closed. It took the therapist som. time to induce the child to make clicks with his mouth open. Then another period of time was necessary to have him produce sounds on exhalation.

To open one's mouth and to speak is to lay oneself bare, and this may be experienced as very dangerous. As a patient of Zeligs (1961) put it:

> Talking to you means revealing myself, which means I'm afraid to reveal my whole self. I have to keep it private, not open to scrutiny or criticism. It's like giving something away, once it's said it can't be taken back. Talking means giving up my identity.

All this suggests that in order to be able to use speech actively in interaction with others, the child has to resolve into a well-balanced synthesis the two antithetic values of speaking, namely aggressiveness and self-exposure. Probably the child must learn to tolerate some degree of aggression towards others and to sustain a certain amount of alien invasion, before he can have normal verbal intercourse with people. In other words, adequate use of speech seems to imply a sufficient structuration of the ego as well as the possibility of an objective relationship. There must be enough self-acceptance and enough willingness to self-disclosure.

Probably, children with selective mutism fail to achieve the necessary level of assertiveness and of openness. Outside of a restricted circle of close relatives they are unable to accept verbal exchange because they lack the assurance which such exchange presupposes. They keep their own counsel in order to be safe from themselves and/or from others.

Their want of self-confidence may be due to various factors, including overprotection by the parents and a mode of education based on excessive conflict avoidance.

It should probably also be recalled that the mouth is sometimes considered a symbol of the vagina. In slang, for instance, the word 'mouth' can be used to denote the female pudenda. The symbolic analogy between the oral and the vaginal cavities underlies the myth of the 'vagina dentata', the toothed vagina. The likening of the mouth to the vagina may possibly contribute to the reluctance of some mute females to open their mouth. Indeed, it may be one of the reasons why selective mutism is more frequent in females than in males.

In Simenon's novel *Le Chat*, Marguerite, after she had declined to have sexual relations with her husband, finally stopped talking to him. Probably in her view sexual intercourse and oral–verbal intercourse implied the same kind of intimacy, which she rejected.

As a matter of fact the resemblance between speaking and making love is perceived as very close by a number of people. For instance, in *Lady Chatterley's Lover*, D.H. Lawrence expressed the view that 'sex is just another form of talk, where you act the words instead of saying them ... Sex might be a sort of normal physical conversation between a man and a woman'.

The word 'conversation' itself points to the relationship between the two actions, as it can be used to refer to verbal exchange as well as to sexual intercourse (especially in the phrase 'criminal conversation', which means 'adulterous relationships') Another example is the word 'abuse' which may denote a verbal as well as a sexual assault. Also 'intercourse' means not only 'communication' but also 'copulation'. Interestingly, this word has a third meaning, 'communion', which seems to form the link between the first two.

Again, according to *Webster's Third New International Dictionary of the English Language*, the phrase 'to be on speaking terms' may denote 'a mutual relationship limited to casual greeting or conversation' as well as 'a mutual relation of intimacy and trust'. According to the same dictionary, 'communication' meant in early days not only 'conversation, talk', but also 'sexual intercourse'.

Because of the resemblance between speaking and making love, speech is likened to sperm. Words are ascribed a creative and generative power. In the beginning God said: 'Let there be light: and there was light.' The word of God created the whole world (Genesis 1: 1–31). And the Blessed Virgin became pregnant after God's representative, the Archangel Gabriel, had told her that she would. The word of God fecundated her (Luke 1: 26–38).

For many people love is inseparable from speech. There can be no true deep sentimental bond without verbal exchange. 'Verba dat omnis amans' Ovid wrote in *Ars Amandi*. Lovers are profuse in words. They talk to each other to maintain and increase their proximity, to commune with each other, to become one. If this unique state of oneness is reached, then speech can be temporarily dropped (see p. 5). But the blessed unity does not last, and speech is resumed to bring and hold the partners together again.

Accordingly, if verbal communication is interrupted, doubts arise as to the continued existence of love, as in the dialogue imagined by Hayakawa (1964, p. 75):

> Wife: Wilbur, why don't you talk to me?
> Husband (interrupted in his reading): What's that?
> Wife: Why don't you talk to me?
> Husband: But there isn't anything to say.
> Wife: You don't love me.

Could it be that the close relationship between speech and love is intuitively perceived by selectively mute children who are possessive and strongly tied to their mother? Could it be that they tend to reserve their speech for their mother because, in a true Oedipean sense, they want to be her lover and do not want to share their love with anyone else, especially not strangers?

Whilst in some selectively mute children suppression of speech may conceivably reflect their exclusive attachment to their mother, in a couple selective mutism seems to proceed mainly from a desire to break a close relationship and at the same time to punish the partner. When speaking is symbolically equated to making love, refusal to speak to one's partner amounts to refraining from being intimately united to him or her. At the same time the partner is debarred from this union. He or she is refused access to the other's body. In this respect, it is probably significant that in Simenon's novel Marguerite informs her husband not only that she will no longer talk to him but also that she wants him to stop talking to her.

Whilst refusing speech, Marguerite accepts communication in writing. In her view, writing does not commit her to her husband the way speaking would do. Written language does not possess the binding power of speech. It does not, in the opinion of many, create a strong bond or an intimate relation. It does not unite the sender to the addressee. It is egocentric, whereas speech is alterocentric. This is why the mute twins described by Wallace (1987) scribbled notes to communicate with their mother. Indeed, these two girls who hardly ever spoke to anyone, wrote diaries, poems, short stories and even novels, which they tried to have published.

Total Mutism

Total mutism, also called 'hysterical mutism', differs from selective mutism in that it is omnipresent: the patient keeps silent everywhere, he speaks to nobody.

Total mutism in individuals with normal language development

Total mutism may be observed in subjects who have developed normal language skills. In such cases, speech is suspended whilst all other verbal abilities remain unabated. Specifically, the patients understand what they are told. If literate, they comprehend written language and can express themselves in writing. In fact, they often use written language to communicate.

On examination, the patients' peripheral speech organs appear intact. In particular, no motor impairment of the oropharyngeal and laryngeal musculature is observed. Actually, speech production is centrally inhibited as a result of psychological problems.

An instance of total mutism in a bright teenager with normal language development was reported in detail by Munford *et al.* (1976). The patient, called Jennifer, was an adopted child. At the age of 4 years she suffered from a throat infection. She began her menses when she was 10 years old. Periods were always accompanied by a sore throat. At the age of 13 Jennifer had a series of severe colds, the symptoms including coughing. One year later she was hospitalised because of persistent cough. Despite medical treatment, no improvement could be achieved. Six months later a thorough lung examination and a neurological examination took place. Both of them were within normal limits. It was noted that coughing did not occur during sleep. Psychotherapy was given, but to no avail. Indeed, the patient soon showed mutism in addition to frequent coughing.

At the age of 17 she had incessant coughing at the rate of 40–50 per minute and she expressed herself exclusively in writing. She could only partially open her mouth, and refrained from eating meat and items like nuts for fear of aspirating them. An operant conditioning therapy, including an extinction procedure and desensitisation, was started. After a few weeks, Jennifer began to talk again but her speech at first consisted of single-word utterances at a barely audible level. At the same time, the cough decreased both in frequency and in volume, until it became a soft clearing of the throat. Eventually, speech returned to normal.

It is probably significant that Jennifer had a history of throat infections. Patients with psychogenic mutism not infrequently report affections of the larynx or respiratory tract. It is as if the weak point has become the breaking point, what the French call 'l'appel d'organe'. For instance, Nicole, who was described by Garoux *et al.* (1982), had had many rhinolaryngological affections since early childhood, and she presented with a first episode of psychogenic mutism immediately following tonsillectomy. During her second episode, she complained in writing about pain in the throat.

In Jennifer's case the cough may have had the same symbolic meaning as the inability to talk or to open one's mouth widely. Just as we cough to expel bodies and thus to prevent them from entering the lower, i.e. innermost, part of the respiratory tract, so closing the mouth and 'shutting up' preclude alien penetration of our bodies.

Probably for the same reason, one of the author's patients with hysterical mutism frequently made noises as if clearing her throat, when she was addressed verbally. In all likelihood, this constant throat clearing was a symbolic way to prevent the words of her partner from entering her body.

Eating problems

In addition to being mute and to coughing constantly, Jennifer was fussy about food.

This is by no means unusual in patients with psychogenic mutism, whether selective or total. For instance, a patient of Russell's (1864) who became functionally mute following the death of her beloved brother, was very slow in swallowing her food. She conceived a dislike for meat and required urging to take proper meals.

The selectively mute boy whom Goll (1979) took into his house, not only did not speak to the members of his foster family but, in addition, refused to eat in their company. Regarding meals, Johnny, an elective mute seen by Pustrom and Speers (1964). showed 'extreme fussiness, choosiness and reduced intake'. Youngerman's (1979) patient 'often refused to eat the regular family meal, demanding that his mother make special foods for him. Frequently she prepared, and he refused, three successive meals'. A young boy with extrafamilial mutism not only remained totally silent in kindergarten but initially also refused to eat anything while in school (Wright *et al.*, 1985). The two selectively mute teenagers described by Kaplan and Escoll (1973) had shown infantile colic and poor feeding followed by vomiting. Later, there were periods of complete food refusal accompanied by wide swings in weight.

Ann, a 12-year-old mute girl observed by Blotcky and Looney (1960), was anorexic, i.e. she showed an abnormal lack of appetite accompanied by a dislike for food. The twins with selective mutism described by Kroppenberg (1987) refused to eat meat or cheese and were fastidious about vegetables and fruit. Laura, the central mute figure of d'Ambrosio's (1970) book, ate very little. June and Jennifer, the two silent twins described by Wallace (1987), often could not bring themselves to eat in the presence of others. And the girl with extrafamilial and later total mutism described by Chethik (1977) 'at times went for many days eating almost nothing'.

There thus appears to exist a symbolic relationship between eating and speaking. In addition to the fact that both activities have the mouth as their main organ, they are felt to imply the acceptance of an interaction between the body and the outer world, an openness, a penetration. It is probably significant, therefore, that the mute patient of Garoux *et al.* (1982) spontaneously started to speak again after she had had gastric aspiration following absorption of drugs in an attempt to kill herself. She explained that although the aspiration had been painful at the time, it had rendered her elated and different.

Russell (1864) reported that his mute patient not only had eating problems, but also could not be easily persuaded to open her mouth and to protrude her tongue, when the physician wanted to examine her larynx. Moreover, the introduction of the laryngeal mirror caused her to sob violently. Probably this woman experienced the opening of her mouth to speak, to eat, or to allow examination of her vocal cords, as something frightening that exposed her innermost self and enabled alien elements to penetrate her body.

This feeling does not occur only in mute patients. Recently at the speech clinic of Ain Sham University in Cairo, Egypt, a Muslim woman with a voice disorder objected to having her larynx examined. Obviously she experienced indirect laryngoscopy as a violation of her inner self.

Opening the mouth to speak may therefore have the same symbolic meaning as opening it to show the speech organs or to take food.

The relationship between eating and speaking may conceivably be enhanced by the existence of a third term, namely making love, which is felt to be akin to either action.

As was shown above, the connection between love and speech is often experienced as a very close one. But the connection between copulating and eating also seems strong. As a matter of fact, quite a number of patients with mental anorexia have a reduced libido, if not an aversion to sex. Anorexic women not infrequently enjoy having become amenorrhoeic, because they find menstruation disgusting. As for obese women, they tend to have menstrual irregularities and to be less fertile than women with a normal weight (Abraham and Llewellyn-Jones, 1984). Also, 'each person's genital odors partly reflect the type of foods they eat' (Masters, Johnson and Kolodny, 1986, p. 314).

There is, then, a bond between loving and taking food. Actually, when we are very fond of somebody, we may feel like eating him or her.

The vocabulary bears testimony to the symbolic link between sexual and feeding behaviours. For instance, in English, 'luscious' may be used in reference to food (= delicious) as well as to a woman (= voluptous, seductive). The adjective 'toothsome' means both 'palatable' (food) and 'sexually attractive'. 'To devour a woman with one's eyes' is to look intently and admiringly at her. 'Morsel' is applicable to a small quantity of food as well as to an attractive girl.

In unconventional English (see Partridge, 1961) 'bite' can be used to denote the female pudenda, and 'biter' to refer to a lascivious girl. The phrase 'to do a bite' may mean 'to eat' or 'to copulate'. 'Suck and swallow' refers to the female, and 'sucker' to the male genitals. 'To eat' is slang for 'to perform cunnilingus'.

In colloquial German, 'jemanden zum Fressen gern haben' (literally: to affection someone to the point of eating him) means 'to be very fond of somebody'.

Of a pretty woman the French say: 'Elle est belle à croquer' (literally: she is so beautiful that you would gobble her). Originally, 'croquer' in this phrase probably meant 'to sketch, to draw', the complete phrase amounting to 'she is as pretty as a picture'. Nowadays, however, people mainly think of 'croquer' as the equivalent of 'to munch'. This is undoubtedly the case in the slang expression 'croquer une poulette' (literally: 'to scrunch a chick'), which means 'to get a girl'. The phrase 'passer à la casserole' (literally: to be cooked in the stewpan) means (of a woman) 'to have undesired sexual intercourse with a man'. A woman who has had many love affairs is called 'mangeuse d'hommes' (literally: man-devourer). 'Appétissant(e)' (literally: appetising) can be said of a dish as well as of a woman.

The English substantive 'agape' also points to the link between eating and loving, as it may be used to denote 'a common meal of fellowship' as well as 'brotherly love' (see *Webster's Third New International Dictionary of the English Language*). The Lord's Supper clearly had this double meaning, and Judas's betrayal was all the more abominable because he had dipped his bread in the dish with Jesus (Matthew 26: 23).

Thus, food and sex, eating and loving, are closely associated. Since taking food and speaking are also interrelated just as love and speech are, it can be said that speaking, making love and eating form an emblematic trilogy. Each of these activities can metaphorically represent the other two.

In this connection, the observations made by Basso (1970) among the Western Apaches are worth mentioning. She found that when they start courting, Apache youngsters 'go without speaking for conspicuous lengths of time'. For hours sweethearts may walk or sit silently side by side.

One of Basso's female informants tried to explain this taciturnity. She reported that her mother had strongly advised her not to be talkative when going out with boys, for eagerness to speak betrays previous experience with men. Indeed, it might at times be interpreted as a willingness to engage in sexual relations.

In pathology speech and sexuality may also be metaphorically associated. For instance, in a case reported by Morgenstein (1927), mutism was found to be tightly linked to the young patient's fear of castration and to his shame of his tendency to masturbation.

One might at this point venture a further consideration. As was shown above, a relationship seems to exist between mutism, particularly selective mutism, and enuresis—encopresis. Although the nature of this relationship is not clear, its existence points to some kind of link between oral—verbal activity and sphincter control.

On the other hand, urination is sometimes associated with copulation. In fact, the two activities to some extent use the same organs. The penis serves both the excretory and the reproductive functions of the body, and the vagina is located close to the urethra (= urinary duct), the pubic labia (lips) forming an entrance to both.

In children's minds coition and micturition are not always clearly differentiated. In adults' symbology, one behaviour may represent the other. For instance, one of Lorenzo Lotto's paintings shows a nude woman (Venus) and by her side, a little boy (Cupid) who is urinating in her direction. His behaviour probably symbolises copulation.

Four actions, then, appear to be interrelated: eating, toileting, copulating and speaking. What have these four body functions in common? Maybe their denominator is that they all have social significance. Each of them establishes a bond between the individual and those around him. They are primary modes of interaction with the environment.

Obviously, eating can be a solitary action. Hermits eat, even though they are alone in the desert. But the primeval act of eating, namely sucking, implies a close relationship between the newborn and his mother, and it creates a strong bond between the two of them.

Later in life, meals taken in common by adults frequently have a social meaning. They bring the participants closer to one another. This is why a banquet is often held at the end of a ceremony or official meeting. Sharing food is regarded as a sign of mutual recognition and reciprocal sympathy.

Bowel and bladder control is also performed primarily out of regard for other people. Natural as it is, the excretory function of the body is socially inconvenient, unless precautions are taken. At Versailles under Louis XIV, courtiers and servants used to urinate and defaecate rather inconsiderately at very many places in and around the castle, and this was a great public nuisance.

As for speaking and making love, they imply a relationship with a partner. These two actions link the participants to one another, and enable them to commune with each other. Significantly, in Allende's novel *The House of the Spirits* (1986), the first sentence spoken by Clara after 9 years of psychogenic silence is to announce that she wants to get married. Clara starts to speak again when she can open up to somebody and can tolerate an intimate relationship with him.

Basically, speaking , eating, making love and toileting foster an objective situation. They help the individual outgrow an initial state of ego-centrism and adapt to social life. They enable him to interact with others and thus to become better aware of both his own personality and the interdependence of the members of the community.

It may be of some significance that the three actions which are related to speaking, namely eating, evacuating and copulating, typify the three stages through which the child is assumed to evolve in early infancy, namely the oral, anal and genital phases of development. This is probably why in his psychodynamic treatment of a mute girl, Chethik (1977) found it desirable to work 'on conflicts related to oral, anal and phallic strivings'.

Amimia

Psychogenic mutism may be accompanied by lack of facial expression, as a case reported by Cummings *et al.* (1983) shows. The patient became suddenly mute at the age of 49 years. He continued to work, but his performance gradually deteriorated and his gait became unsteady. He progressively withdrew from social contact. At the same time he started to show great concern about his bowels. When aged 54 he stopped eating and was for this reason admitted to hospital. For the first few days following admission, the patient had abdominal pain and watery diarrhoea. He did not eat. He was delusional and claimed in writing to be on a diet. After several days of intravenous hydration, nasogastric tube feeding and treatment with antipsychotic agents, he resumed eating,

The patient understood speech normally and expressed himself in writing. He did not speak at all. In addition, he was amimic. He had no spontaneous facial expression and was unable to pantomime emotions. Neither could he grunt, hum, cough or yawn on request. Moving the tongue on order was slow. On the other hand, there was no dysphagia. The gag reflex was increased. Indirect laryngoscopy disclosed no laryngeal pathology.

The patient had difficulty in moving his gaze upward on request and in pursuit of an object. Tone was increased. Gait was narrow based with short, shuffling steps. The patient's posture was midly bowed. Neuropsychological assessment pointed to some mental regression. There was marked depression and anxiety, with numerous somatic concerns and some delusional ideation.

Initial treatment with antipsychotic drugs was replaced by antidepressant therapy. The patient's depression and amimia decreased. He could now cough softly on request. But he remained totally mute.

Gradual vs sudden onset

In some cases total mutism sets in gradually or even insidiously. Not infrequently, it is ushered in by aphonia, i.e. absence of voice. For some time, the patient speaks in a whisper and then completely ceases to communicate orally. For instance, Mary, a young patient observed by Straughan (1986), started to whisper instead of producing voiced speech, after her mother had reprimanded her at 3 years of age. The girl became withdrawn and a few weeks later ceased to speak altogether.

Following the extraction of 18 teeth in two sittings, a patient of Rugg (1887) lost her voice. For a year and a half she was unable to speak above a whisper. Then she became totally mute.

In other cases, total mutism is preceded by selective mutism. As an instance, the case of Anna reported by Goll (1979) may be quoted. The girl did not start to speak until she was 4 years old. Then she started to use speech at home, but would remain completely silent whenever strangers were present. She never spoke outside her home.

At the age of 7 Anna was put in an institution and later in a foster family. She learned to read and write but became totally mute. Even during visits to her biological parents, she would not talk. However, she regularly wrote to her father, to whom she seemed to be greatly attached.

Another instance of gradual onset of mutism was reported by Dugas *et al.* (1972). Their patient, a 7.5-year-old boy, first ceased to speak to, or in the presence of, his father. A little later his mutism became total. The same progression was observed in the case reported by Morgenstern (1927).

Occasionally, total mutism is ushered in by an anomalous verbal behaviour different from aphonia or selective mutism. For instance, Ajuriaguerra, Diaktine and de Gobineau (1956) briefly described a schoolgirl with behavioural disorders who at the age of 8 started to use neologisms to denote relatives. She would become angry when these neo-formations were not readily understood but would not let other people use them. A little later, psychogenic mutism set in. The patient communicated in writing, sometimes profusely. Some of her messages were written mirror fashion.

At times, however, there are no forerunners and total mutism begins abruptly. For example, Gilles, a 4-year-old boy described by Kohler and Vuagnat (1971), became suddenly and totally mute after he had been laughed at by his classmates because he had wetted himself two times in succession.

Total mutism began suddenly also in a case reported by Schachter (1967). The patient, a girl of almost 4 years, was involved in a traffic accident which, in addition to causing a few superficial wounds, left the child totally mute for 4 days. For the first 2 days after the accident there was also enuresis and on one occasion encopresis. No neurological signs could be observed.

After 4 days speech gradually returned, but the girl, who used to speak fluently, now had a rather severe stutter with initial sound repetitions and, in polysyllabic words, initial syllable repetitions. Stuttering lasted for 6 months.

Reluctant speech

In some cases, mutism is not absolute. From time to time, the patient reacts briefly to a question or possibly says something of his own accord. He is therefore considered to have reluctant speech or to be reticent.

Two teenagers with reluctant speech were described by Kaplan and Escoll (1973). The patients were reticent and depressive girls who used speech very sparingly and, at times, even totally refrained from speaking, especially when addressed by their own father.

Generally, reticent individuals lack conversational assertiveness. They are apprehensive of playing an active role in oral communication. They see themselves as inept in verbal interaction, and seem to think that it is better to remain silent and let people think you are a fool than to speak and prove it to them.

Kaplan and Escoll (1973) considered that in their two cases one of the reasons why the father was not spoken to was the girls' unconscious desire not to come too close to their father to whom they, in fact, felt sexually attracted.

Mutism in battle stress casualties

In war time functional mutism is sometimes observed in soldiers who have experienced intense fear on the battle field. These soldiers may have gone through a heavy bombardment or have sustained a fierce attack which probably killed several of their companions. They themselves may have been blown up or wounded. They may have lain unconscious for some time after the shelling.

An officer who during World War I went through such a frightful experience related it as follows:

> My nerves were strung up to such a pitch that I felt that something in me would snap. Every shell fired seemed to be nearer the mark than the last, and the ground all around was covered with shell holes. The general feeling was that 'the next one' would land right in the post. Part of the trench had already been blown in. The back blast from each explosion flattened us up against the wall of the trench. (Brown, 1918)

Mutism in battle stress casualties may appear immediately after the dreadful experience or a few hours or even a few days later. It may be the only deficit or, on the contrary, be accompanied by functional deafness or by functional paralysis of the extremities.

Initially, it may be difficult to distinguish this hysterical mutism from real aphasic disorders, especially if the patient has suffered a head wound which may conceivably have disturbed cerebral language mechanisms.

Signs which may help the clinician arrive at a correct diagnosis are the presence of functional motor or sensory disorders, the presence of stupor or apathy and the absence of written language disturbances. Generally such signs are not encountered in aphasic patients, i.e. in patients whose verbal disorders are directly caused by organic brain damage.

Dynamics of total mutism

Luria (1970, pp. 43–44) expressed the view that functional mutism, and even more so mutism accompanied by functional deafness, is in fact a defence mechanism. Having to sustain unbearable stress, the individual retreats into a protective shell of silence. His mutism, possibly reinforced by his deafness, encapsulates him and thus enables him to withdraw from a world of horror that can no longer be coped with.

In other cases, silence enables a break with an environment that can no longer be trusted or loved. It builds a refuge from the outside world and disconnects the patient from those around him. It enables him to withdraw into a transparent but waterproof cocoon. The person with total mutism is present but inaccessible. After a spell of mutism, a patient of Abraham and Llewellyn-Jones (1984, p. 88) indicated that by keeping silent she had constructed 'an impermeable barrier' around herself. And she added: 'I couldn't cope outside of it.'

Speech establishes a direct relation between the partners. Specifically, it commits the speaker to his listener. By remaining silent, the patient avoids this personal engagement, this consignment of himself to another person.

Also, silence can guard the individual from disappointment, for, if we do not speak and consequently never ask for anything, we cannot incur rejection, we cannot be denied or turned down. Tolentino's (1957) patient who had spells of total mutism alternating with spells of selective mutism, wrote to her psychiatrist:

> I do not speak, I do not disturb you, I do not ask you for anything. I have no desire, I do not want to have any desire. I only take what you give me, what is within my reach. In this manner I take nothing away from anybody. Nobody can hurt me, because I do not compete with anyone; I do not fight against anyone to get something.

Even after she had conquered her mutism, d'Ambrosio's (1970) patient Laura often refrained from asking for something, lest her request should not be accepted. For instance, she abstained from asking her therapist to attend the graduation ceremony at her high school, because she was afraid he might not acquiesce to her request. After the ceremony, she explained to d'Ambrosio that she preferred to keep thinking that he might have accepted, had she asked, than to run the risk of incurring a refusal.

Silence may also give the individual the impression that he is powerful and can control himself and his environment. In her written notes to her psychiatrist, Tolentino's (1957) patient indicated that she did not express her resentment in order to let it grow within herself. If she had put it in words, it would have dissipated and lost its strength. Because it had not been expressed, her resentment was intact and fully potent. The patient felt like an ominous gunpowder barrel that could explode and blast her environment. The less she said, the fuller she felt. She was rich from all the words she had not spoken. She hoarded speech as a miser hoards gold.

Also, by refraining from talking about herself and her feelings, Tolentino's patient left her environment in doubt as to her real state of mind. People around her could therefore hardly affect her. The patient felt that she thus had better control over them.

Indeed, by keeping completely silent, patients may feel that they inflict pain on others and thus can punish them. Several observations, including those of Garoux et al. (1982), show that mutes may be perfectly aware of this way to torment those around them.

However, mutism may also result from a desire to control and even to repress one's own aggression. The patient keeps his mouth shut lest he should strike out at the others. Hayden (1983) described an adolescent with long-standing mutism and many phobias. When treatment succeeded in removing the mutism and discarding the fears, the patient appeared exceedingly aggressive and full of hatred.

As for the patient of Garoux et al. (1982), when she recovered speech, she did not want to be discharged from the hospital and to go home, because she was afraid of what she might do to her relatives. She said that she could abuse them or even beat them. When some time later she did return to her family, she had a fight with her mother and another with her brother (who had told her to shut up!).

Prognosis and therapy

If left untreated, total mutism may eventually clear up spontaneously. In some cases, the cause of this spontaneous recovery remains obscure. For instance, a woman described by Rugg (1887) had had total mutism for more than 3 years and regained her speech one day, but the reasons for this spontaneous recovery were not clear.

In other instances, the recovery although unexpected can be better explained. For instance, the patient of Garoux et al. (1982) started to speak again after she had had gastric aspiration (see p. 43).

Spontaneous recovery was also observed in some battle stress casualties. At times, however, only articulation returned. The patient spoke in a whisper. This whispered speech could be halting and require visible efforts to be produced. In other soldiers, mutism spontaneously evolved into stammering.

However, rather than clearing up, total mutism may persist and become a permanent component of the patient's make-up. Critchley (1970, p. 387) reported on a young woman who became mute when she was 5 or 6 years old. Despite her speechlessness she went through school, having answered all the teachers' questions in writing or by means of finger spelling. Later she was able to take and hold down a job in a factory. She was courted by a young man who eventually married her.

In addition to being mute, she had hypomimia, i.e. her face was barely expressive. The noise she made when coughing, laughing, sneezing or weeping was extremely subdued. In her sleep she at times made moaning noises. She had a pet budgerigar to which she would occasionally make little sounds. Once in a while, when pressed, she would whisper a short answer.

As an adult she was followed up for several years. No significant change was observed in her verbal behaviour during this period. She had always declined to be taken for therapy.

For patients who, in contradistinction to this woman, are willing to be treated several therapeutic procedures are available.

Some clinicians apply psychodynamic techniques. When the patient is young, these techniques consist mainly in interpreting play or drawing and connecting them with past or present conflicts. As an example the case described by Morgenstern (1927) may be quoted. The patient was a boy who 2 years previously had had an episode of psychogenic mutism lasting a few weeks. One year before examination he ceased to speak to his father. Eight months later complete mutism set in again.

When first examined he was totally mute but answered yes–no questions by nodding his head. It was decided to give him therapy.

As he liked drawing, he was encouraged to produce drawings and to answer questions graphically. His productions were taken to indicate that he was terribly afraid of his father and suffered from a castration complex. By interpreting the drawings in a manner which the child could understand, the therapist managed to eliminate the fears and to reinstate active speech.

When the patient is a child, the therapist may deem it desirable to give the parents concomitant counselling. At times, he may even recommend them for psychotherapy.

Case reports of mute children treated psychodynamically often mention the manifestation of aggressiveness, and sometimes also of regressive behaviour, during therapy. These abreactions are accepted by the therapist, as they are assumed to have a cathartic effect and to favour the return of speech.

At times, when mutism is of recent occurrence and is not accompanied by psychological disturbances, suggestion may be sufficient to re-establish a normal verbal behaviour. Wallis (1957) briefly mentioned a teenager who suddenly became speechless while she was being scolded by her father for returning late from a surprise party. Her mutism could easily be cured through persuasion.

In some cases, suggestion is used after the patient has been given an injection of barbiturate or of amphetamine.

Suggestion may also take place under hypnosis. Brown (1918) used this method with British battle stress casualties. He would induce a slight hypnotic sleep in the patient and tell him that he was going to experience again the frightening situation which had rendered him speechless. Usually this caused the patient to become restless and after a few seconds to start shouting and to pantingly relate the terrifying event he had gone through at the front. The soldier thus abreacted the violent emotion which had brought on mutism. He was then slowly awakened and asked to remember what had happened during sleep. When fully conscious he would recall having talked during hypnosis, and this enabled him to overcome his mutism.

Hirschfeld (1916) used a different method in the German army. He would inform the mute patient that he was going to apply a faradic current to his throat in an effort to deblock the speech mechanism. The patient was to shout if the current was too strong. A rather strong current was then applied. Invariably, Hirschfeld reported, the patient screamed. This made him realise that his speech organs could function. He could then easily be induced to talk normally.

Bittorf (1915), who applied the same method, contended that fright engendered by the electric current terminated mutism just as fright on the battle field started it.

Muck (1917) used to elicit a fright reaction in mute patients by introducing a foreign body, shaped like a bullet, into their glottis. The patients had the impression that they were going to choke and reacted with a powerful exhalation accompanied by a cry. After that, they could easily be persuaded to talk again.

A similar approach had already been used by Bach (1890) at the end of the nineteenth century. He described his technique as follows:

> The greatest difficulty with the hysterical patient is the production of the first tone, as such patients are generally unable, through their own efforts, to produce any sound whatsoever. The initial difficulty, however, can always be overcome in a few moments by the assistance of reflex action. For this purpose, a strong irritant, whether mechanical or chemical, may be applied to the larynx so as to excite the cough. This of course requires no effort on the part of the patient. Having excited this cough once or twice the patient will be able to reproduce it independently of the irritant ... It now becomes a simple matter to continue this cough and to pronounce, more or less distinctly, the vowel 'a' at each effort and after a few

efforts to substitute the vowel 'e', and so on, until all the vowels have been coughed. After this is repeated several times, the elements of cough can easily be eliminated from the vocalisation, when we have left the pure vowel-sounds, which, without effort on the part of the patient, can be combined with consonants ... first placing the vowel before the consonant and then reversing this. It would not be advisable to attempt the articulation of words at this stage, but better to combine the vowels with single consonants, gradually increasing the duration of the sound. The patient is thus led to speak words without resisting, wilfully or unintentionally.

Simple as they are, these mechanical methods may not be harmless in cases where functional mutism reflects a deeply rooted relational problem. If this problem is not treated, mutism may possibly disappear but it is likely to be replaced by another symptom which can be even more incapacitating.

Can mutism be suddenly cured by a strong affect?

As was mentioned above, Hirschfeld (1916), Bittorf (1915) and, most of all, Muck (1917) deliberately resorted to fright to deblock the inhibited speech mechanisms of their mute patients. The clients' panic resulted from a direct physical aggression sustained by their larynx. Can fear also put a sudden end to mutism when it is not related to the larynx or when the patient's body is not touched? And can other strong emotions have the same effect?

An ancient legend has it that Croesus, the wealthy king of Lydia, had a son who had never spoken. One day the boy witnessed a frightening scene: a soldier was about to slaughter his father. Horrified the child shouted: 'Soldier, don't kill Croesus'. From that moment he could speak (*Herodotus I*, 85).

This story implies that horror can cure an individual of his functional mutism. However, the medical literature does not seem to contain reports of psychogenic mutism suddenly terminated by fear. A dreadful sight can undoubtedly strike someone dumb but it is uncertain whether it can heal mutism. Despite fictions to the contrary, it does not seem possible to frighten someone out of his speechlessness.

Mutism in schizophrenics

As mutism is a way to avoid close association with others and for an individual to insulate himself, it is not surprisingly encountered in a number of schizophrenics. Some of them are completely silent, whilst others do not use speech to communicate but can from time to time be heard to mumble to themselves. For instance, Isaacs, Thomas and Goldiamond (1960) reported on a 40-year-old catatonic schizophrenic man who had been mute for 19 years. An operant conditioning therapy with chewing gum as a tangible reinforcer was used in an attempt to re-establish some speech behaviour. After a few weeks a situation resembling selective mutism could be brought about. The patient would answer his therapist's questions but would speak to no one else. The therapy was continued and eventually the patient started to answer a particular nurse's questions also. From then on, he from time to time briefly talked to other people.

Another schizophrenic patient had been mute for 14 years. Following behaviour modification therapy, this situation slightly improved. The patient would now answer questions during group therapy sessions. Elsewhere he remained totally silent.

In 1963 Sherman described a 53-year-old paranoid schizophrenic who in the course of the last 26 years had been heard to talk only once. On that particular occasion he had made a two-word reply to a ward attendant's question. For the rest, the patient had been completely mute. However, he would communicate in writing both spontaneously and in reaction to questions. This written communication was limited to the ward attendants. The patient never wrote notes meant for other inmates.

Through operant conditioning this man could be brought to gradually substitute nods, grunts and finally spoken words for his written messages. Despite his long silence, he was able to speak distinctly and appropriately but in a soft voice.

A few years later, Sherman (1968) wrote about another schizophrenic who had been mute for 16 years. Behaviour modification therapy was started. After some 45 sessions the patient would regularly answer common questions with sentences comprising up to six words.

Another patient described by Sherman (1968) had not used speech for 45 years. A lengthy operant conditioning therapy succeeded in slightly reducing this mutism of long standing. During sessions, the patient could finally be made to name a number of common objects or drawings held up by the examiner and to read aloud his name and the numbers from 1 to 20. However, it is not recorded that he ever could be persuaded to use speech again for communicative purposes.

As may be seen, therapy for mutism in schizophrenic patients often has to be extended over a long period of time before any improvement can be achieved. Moreover, at times the improvement remains limited.

Mutism may be present not only in chronic schizophrenics, but also in individuals who are going through an acute psychotic spell. Akhtar and Buckman (1977) briefly mentioned a patient who was brought in lying flaccidly on a stretcher. His eyes were closed. He was mute and did not follow verbal commands. He responded to painful stimuli by grimacing. Neurological and neuroradiological examination failed to disclose any underlying organic pathology. The next day, the patient suddenly became agitated and physically assaultive, and had to be sedated. Following this he started to talk freely. He recalled the events of the preceding 24 hours. He displayed a flat affect and had complex delusions. A diagnosis of schizophrenia was made. The patient was put on phenotiazines and improved rapidly. He could be discharged 2 weeks later.

Mutism may in fact accompany various behavioural and thought disturbances such as mania and depression. It is a regular component of catatonic episodes. During such spells, patients tend to remain immobile and mute, whilst their consciousness is generally preserved.

Mutism in psychotic children

Psychotic children may also present with complete mutism. In some cases, the child fails to develop expressive speech. He demonstrates speech comprehension but remains mute. In other cases, he begins to speak but later stops using speech actively.

Ajuriaguerra (1977, p. 360) notes that mute children with severe psychosis can sometimes be taught to express themselves in writing. Apparently they experience written language as less binding and, hence, less dangerous than speech.

If treated the child may eventually start to speak (again) but his speech is likely to be hesitant at first. For some time, he will be groping for the correct words, the correct pronunciation and the appropriate vocal pitch.

As an instance of functional mutism in a psychotic child the case related by d'Ambrosio (1970) may be quoted. The patient, Laura, was a 12-year-old girl who as a baby had been beaten and severely burnt by her alcoholic parents. She had been admitted to the hospital in a critical state. After her wounds had finally healed, she was institutionalised. She grew into a sullen and listless girl who never spoke.

D'Ambrosio undertook to treat her. For more than 2 years he tried to involve her in some kind of activity or exchange, to elicit a response. But the girl would stay aloof, immured in her silence. Her therapist had the impression of talking to a brick wall. Finally, using puppets, he staged a dreadful scene in which two parents maltreated their baby. This revival deblocked Laura who started to shout. After this breakthrough, normal use of speech could be progressively established.

Total mutism in individuals with underdeveloped language skills

Complete or nearly complete mutism may also be encountered in individuals with underdeveloped language skills. These patients have limited expressive abilities and for psychological reasons cannot be made to use the little speech they possess. Indeed, they may evidence a negative attitude towards speech and resist any attempt to have them utter words.

This condition is sometimes observed in rejected or maltreated children. For instance, Werner (1945) observed a 5-year-old girl who had never talked. Indeed, according to her father, she had never been heard to utter a sound. She was an unwanted child, largely rejected, or at least ignored, by her mother, who gave her minimum attention and hardly ever talked to her.

At 5 years of age, the patient was a thin, weak and undernourished child. Her comprehension of spoken language was fairly good but she herself never spoke. When urged to speak, she would hide her head, withdraw herself or run away. Her non-verbal behaviour in everyday situations was not suggestive of mental handicap.

Individual speech therapy was initiated. At first the child was persuaded to repeat meaningless sounds produced by the teacher. For instance, the teacher would drop an object and say 'boom' and then would entice the little girl to imitate her.

Through similar play situations other sounds were stimulated. Games were played with toy animals, and a specific sound was associated with each animal. Gradually real words were introduced. The young patient repeated them provided they were monosyllabic. Polysyllabic words were either ignored or abbreviated.

After some time, the child started to name pictures of objects. However, her rendition of the words was often defective or simplified. Moreover, she showed at first no inclination to use her vocabulary outside the word-calling game. But a little later, she became more spontaneous and started to volunteer some simple words in reference to specific items in her home.

Therapy was continued and eventually the child could be made to use disyllables. After some time she could be persuaded to use phrases and to form sentences. She also started to use speech for true communicative purposes.

A year and a half after speech therapy had begun her pronunciation, though understandable, was far from being correct. Word endings were often omitted. Her command of syntax was also defective. Her sentences were frequently incomplete. Despite these verbal shortcomings her negative attitude towards speech had disappeared.

In such a case, it is not easy to decide whether mutism and withdrawal caused the language delay by preventing the child from acquiring linguistic skills through practise or, on the contrary, whether the child refrained from expressing herself orally because she could not do so adequately. In other words, it is not clear whether the negative attitude towards speech was antecedent to or, on the contrary, consequent upon language acquisition difficulties. Possibly psychological, educational and neuro-biological factors interacted to bring about the pathological condition.

Such interplay seems to have been present in a case reported by Adams and Glassner (1954). Their patients were a 9-year-old girl and her 6-year-old brother. Neither of them used language actively.

Their births had been without complications and their motor and psychomotor development had been normal, but for expressive speech. Verbal comprehension was age appropriate and, on examination, no audiological or neurological sign was detected.

The patients' father was a World War I veteran who had developed while in the service, after he had been gassed. His speech had returned a few months later upon arrival in the USA. He was a tyrant at home and, when under the influence of alcohol, demanded absolute silence.

The two children were given intensive speech therapy, but to little avail. Eventually they were placed in a school for the deaf, where they learned to express themselves through gestures and in writing.

When re-examined at the age of 20, the girl was found to have become a dull, inhibited adult with very little, garbled speech. On psychometric testing she achieved a mental age of 16 and an IQ of 87.

Her brother performed at a higher level psychometrically, attaining a mental age of nearly 16 and an IQ of 106. His speech was somewhat more copious than his sister's but equally difficult to understand.

An EEG performed at the time was borderline in the case of the girl and slightly abnormal in her brother's case. It was felt that organic factors must have combined with emotional and environmental ones to produce the patients' persistent reticence.

Individuals who despite underdeveloped verbal skills do use speech to communicate may become mute if their limited linguistic capacities are mocked or criticised. Arnold (1948, pp. 206–208) reported the case of an uneducated labourer with a developmental speech and language impairment. The articulatory difficulties of this man increased after he was involved in a car accident which upset him without causing any organic damage. He was in the army at the time. One day he was rebuked by a superior for his slurred speech. Following this reproof he became totally mute and functionally deaf.

Mutism may also be triggered off by a situation which the patient finds utterly unpleasant or to which he cannot adapt. Launay and Borel-Maisonny (1972, p. 294) reported the case of a schoolgirl from a poor family who had always had deficient language. At 7 years of age, she was sent to a holiday camp which she disliked and where she became totally mute. She was put in a rehabilitation centre where psychotherapy and speech therapy were attempted but without result. She communicated by gestures but avoided looking face to face. When she was nearly 12 years old, psychodynamic therapy based on drawing and later on written language was given. Eventually, speech returned but proved very deficient. It improved somewhat in ensuing years.

In these two cases limited verbal command caused a lack of conversational assertiveness. Under stress the poorly developed verbal ability totally disintegrated.

Conclusions

A number of people fail to exhibit the verbal behaviour which is expected of them: they do not use speech spontaneously or in answer to questions in situations where it is considered appropriate to be verbal. However, they demonstrate normal or at least appreciable speech comprehension. They are therefore said to have mutism.

Their mutism is diagnosed as functional or psychogenic when no lesion or organic disease can be discovered that can reasonably be held to be the cause of the absence of speech.

Some people with functional mutism never speak. Their mutism is total. As regards this complete absence of speech, no difference is observed between children and adults.

Other individuals use speech only with a limited number of partners or, on the contrary, refrain from talking to just one specific person or a limited group of persons. Whilst the former behaviour is typically observed in children, the latter is more frequent among adults. Selective mutism therefore varies in scope according to whether it occurs in children or in adults.

Although different, selective mutism and total mutism have a number of features in common. Moreover, selective mutism may evolve into total mutism or alternate with it.

Not infrequently, mutism is accompanied by other symptoms which also testify to a lack of adaptation to relational life. Examination of these symptoms shows further that there is often felt to exist a close symbolic relationship between speaking, eating, toileting and making love.

Except for selective mutism in adults, mutism is usually considered a detrimental behaviour. It is held to be an obstacle to social integration, to academic achievement and to professional pursuits. At times, as in the case of chronic schizophrenics, it is thought to hinder improvement. For these various reasons, it is regarded as an affection deserving treatment. It is thought to prevent the individual from entering fully into possession of his human inheritance. As a consequence, society feels entitled, and in duty bound, to try to eliminate it. The possibility that the patient might be more happy as a silent individual, or might feel more comfortable if he does not speak, is not usually considered.

Patients with psychogenic mutism are generally given behaviour modification therapy or psychotherapy, or a combination of the two. At times, suggestion and hypnosis are also resorted to.

The outcome of therapy is variable, depending, it would seem, on the personality of the mute patient, the reasons why he keeps silent and the way his problem is approached.

Chapter 4
The Syndrome of Mutism: Organic Mutism

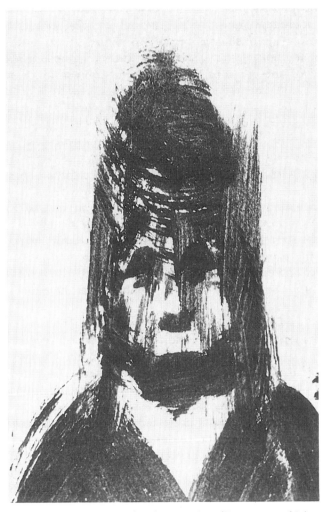

Figure 2. Self-portrait by a patient with aphasic mutism. (By courtesy of Jolanta W. and Maria Pachalska.)

Introductory Remarks

The notion of organicity

Patients are considered to have organic mutism when an organic lesion can be demonstrated that may be reasonably held to be responsible for the absence of expressive speech, or else when there is no apparent psychological problem and the absence of oral–verbal expression is accompanied by other deficits equally suggestive of an affection or dysfunction of the central nervous system.

The diagnosis of organic mutism is not always easy to make and there are cases where the organicity of the condition may be questioned. As an instance of disputable diagnosis, the case reported by Cummings *et al.* (1983) and mentioned on p. 46 may be quoted. The authors considered that their patient's mutism was organic in nature and 'was the result of lesions involving both limbic system and descending neocortical connections'. However, these lesions could not be unequivocally demonstrated. In fact, the skull roentgenograms and an EEG were normal, whilst computerised tomography showed but slight widening of the sylvian fissures, an enlarged third ventricle and slight dilatation of the left lateral ventricle. Whilst not incompatible with the assumption of lesions affecting the limbic system and the neocortical areas and their descending connections, these findings certainly do not prove the assumption to be correct.

In fact, the patient showed a number of symptoms that are usually indicative of brain pathology, such as increased tone, narrow-based gait, asymmetrical stretch reflexes and limited volitional upgaze. In all probability, the patient had some affection of the central nervous system. It is not sure, however, whether this disease was the cause of the speech suppression. In other words, it may be doubted that the patient's mutism was organic.

As a matter of fact, the patient had been mute for 5 years. During this period he had progressively withdrawn from social contact and had become preoccupied with somatic concerns. In the final few months before hospitalisation his behaviour deteriorated. His admission was precipitated when he stopped eating. All this is certainly compatible with the notion of psychologically based mutism.

The patient resumed eating after he had been given antipsychotic drugs for a few days. As the Minnesota Multiphasic Personality Inventory (MMPI) profile demonstrated marked depression and anxiety with numerous somatic concerns and some delusional ideation, the initial treatment was replaced by antidepressant therapy. This brought about an improvement of the patient's general condition and of his amimia. This man, then, had serious psychological problems, which could be somewhat reduced pharmacologically.

Cummings *et al.* (1983) assumed that their patient's mutism and lack of facial expression were due to an intracranial cerebrovascular disease with multiple small lacunar infarctions in the internal capsules and deep nuclear structures adjacent to the third ventricle. However, there was no neuroradiological evidence to support this assumption. Moreover, it is surprising that bilateral infarctions in the internal capsules should have caused total paralysis of the speech musculature but no chewing and swallowing difficulties. Usually, bilateral injury to the corticobulbar tracts in the internal capsules entail dysphagia in addition to problems with speech production (see pp. 70 and 73).

It may therefore be doubted whether, in the case reported by Cummings *et al.* (1983), mutism was organic in nature.

This example shows that the distinction between functional and organic mutism is not always easy to make.

In some cases, the decision depends on the opinion that is held concerning the nature of the syndrome of which mutism is a component. For instance, the absence of expressive speech in some autistic children will be considered organic or, on the contrary, functional, depending on whether autism is held to be an organic disorder or a psychosis.

When an organic lesion is found that can legitimately be considered responsible for the speech suppression, this does not always make an explanation of the observed mutism possible. As will be seen in connection with akinetic mutism (see p. 93) and with mutism accompanied by a pyramidal hemisyndrome (see p. 78), the discovery of the causal lesion does not always enable an account to be made for the loss of speech. The pathophysiology of the speechlessness may be unclear, even though the cerebral injury responsible for it has been located. In other words, we cannot always understand why the cerebral damage suffered by the patient has rendered him mute. The pathogenesis may remain elusive in the face of obvious brain insult.

Types of organic mutism

Organic mutism may result from injury to the peripheral speech organs as well as from damage to the central nervous system. A distinction is therefore usually made between organic mutism of peripheral origin and organic mutism of central origin.

The central lesion responsible for the absence of speech may be congenital or neonatal and, as such, may prevent the development of speaking skills. The resultant mutism is then said to be developmental.

If, on the contrary, damage to the central nervous system is incurred after the individual has learned to speak, and causes the loss of the ability to use speech expressively, the ensuing mutism is called 'acquired'.

Theoretically, a distinction can also be made between developmental and acquired peripheral mutism. However, as will be seen presently, this distinction has little practical value.

Mutism of Peripheral Origin

Laryngectomy

Mutism following classic laryngectomy is a typical example of peripherally based mutism. In patients undergoing classic laryngectomy, the oral–pharyngeal cavity is completely disconnected from the lower part of the respiratory tract. The patient breathes through a tracheostoma, which is an opening made by the surgeon in the neck a few centimetres above the sternum. Through the tracheostoma air is directly inhaled into the trachea and lungs.

The pharynx is completely severed from the trachea in order to avoid aspiration during eating and drinking. As a result, no egressive air can pass from the trachea to the oral–pharyngeal cavity, and no audible speech can be produced.

Distress

Most laryngectomees experience speech deprivation as an utterly distressing situation. Although they can express themselves in writing, they find the inability to speak highly depressant. They have the crushing feeling of having been bereft of something typically human and essential to the quality of life. They are dummies in the double sense of the word: mute and sham. The American actor William Gargan (1969, p. 240) recalled that immediately after laryngectomy he felt as worthless as an old silent film: 'The silent movies were dead. So, in a sense, was I.'

At times, the silent laryngectomee's despair is so great that it overrides religious conviction. Although he was a devout Catholic, one of the author's laryngectomised patients attempted twice to commit suicide because he could not resign himself to being mute. He explained in writing that those who can speak have no idea of the abysmal desperation to which speechlessness can drive a person.

De Bruine Groeneveldt (1924) described a laryngectomee who killed himself because he could not live without speech. Barton (1965) mentioned two patients whose larynges he had had to remove. Out of despair one of them committed suicide and the other took to drinking.

Speech rehabilitation

Fortunately, a number of techniques are available which enable laryngectomees to speak again.

Many patients learn to use their oesophagus to produce voice and an egressive air stream. A muscular constriction which they bring about at the base of their pharynx replaces the lost vocal cords.

Generally, oesophageal speech requires months of training and exercises before it is fully mastered. Moreover, the voice of the oesophageal speaker is usually raucous and low pitched. Still, many clinicians advise their laryngectomised patients to try to acquire oesophageal speech because it is a form of speech produced entirely by the body; it is not dependent on any mechanical device; it is available to the patient at any time and it is entirely organic and therefore can be fairly easily incorporated into the patient's image of self, at least in the case of male laryngectomees. Because it is low pitched, oesophageal voice is sometimes less acceptable to females.

The acquisition and use of oesophageal speech can be facilitated by the placement of a tracheo-oesophageal valve by the surgeon. Through this valve pulmonary air can be directed into the oesophagus, from where it can be expelled towards the oropharyngeal cavity. This system generally enables the patient to speak louder and to form longer sentences in one breath than in ordinary oesophageal speech. Moreover, the patient need not learn to aspirate air into his oesophagus. On the other hand, the tracheo-oesophageal valve has to be replaced every now and then, and it may get clogged.

Some surgeons reconstruct a meatus between the trachea and the pharynx and provide the upper end of it with folds which can be used as a neoglottis. This neoglottis is activated by air from the lungs as in normal speakers. However, this organic valve is not always completely foolproof. At times, liquids seep through it, causing violent cough.

Finally, laryngectomees can speak by means of an artificial larynx, which may be pneumatic or electronic. Various models exist (Lebrun, 1973) and generally they are easy to use, requiring little or no practice. On the other hand, they are conspicuous. Moreover, the patient is totally dependent on his prosthesis to produce speech. If the artificial larynx is broken, lost or simply not at hand, the laryngectomee cannot express himself orally.

Glossectomy

Mutism as it is observed in adults who have undergone laryngectomy may meaningfully be considered a form of acquired mutism of peripheral origin. Morphological changes brought about in the peripheral speech organs result in the inability to produce audible speech. Speaking skills are lost following surgical removal of the larynx.

Sometimes, another part of the vocal tract has to be excised, namely the tongue. Although this organ is the main articulator, its removal does not generally render the patient mute. To begin with, the glossectomy d s not interfere with phonation. Moreover, once their surgical wounds have healed, glossectomees usually prove able to produce speech (compare Goldstein, 1940; Skelly *et al.*, 1971; La Riviere, Seilo and Dimmick, 1975; Morrish, 1988). In fact, their articulation is grossly deviant and intelligibility is reduced. With practice articulation may improve, reaching at times an astonishing degree of comprehensibility. In other cases, it remains difficult to understand, despite the patient's efforts to speak more clearly. In virtually no case is the patient really speechless, but some glossectomees refrain from speaking because they are ashamed of the poor quality of their articulation. Pettygrove (1985) has given an autobiographical account of this embarrassment.

Stories have been written in which the tongue of a character is cut to prevent him from speaking. For instance, in the novel *The World According to Garp*, Irving tells about a girl, Ellen James, who was raped by two men. After their misdeed the rapists cut off the victim's tongue in order to prevent her from telling anyone who they were or what they looked like. Irving further relates that to protest at what happened to Ellen James, a number of women had their tongues cut off. They could no longer speak and expressed themselves in writing.

However, clinical cases do not fully bear out such fictions. Speech is possible without tongue, although articulation is always distorted.

Congenital malformations of the vocal tract

A number of fictional works depict characters who never learned to talk because of some congenital defect of the vocal tract. This malformation sometimes consists of the adherence of the tongue to the floor of the mouth (ankyloglossia) or of the lack of development of the tongue (lingual agenesis). Again, clinical observations do not confirm these fictions. In fact, some children are born with severe malformations of the oropharyngeal cavity which, if left untreated, might conceivably preclude the acquisition of speaking skills. But these malformations are usually surgically repaired, or at least amended, because they severely interfere with feeding. As a consequence of the operation(s), speech is usually possible, but articulation may be gravely distorted. In particular, there may be strong hyperrhinolalia (nasal speech).

It follows that apart from laryngectomy, mutilation or malformation of the vocal tract does not generally result in the total absence of oral–verbal expression. However, there may conceivably be exceptions to this rule, especially in countries where no paediatric surgery can be performed.

Deaf–muteness

'Deaf–muteness' is used to refer to a condition in which the absence of hearing has prevented the individual from acquiring both speech comprehension and expressive speech. As such, this condition falls outside the scope of the present book, which considers only cases where speech comprehension is normal or largely present, whilst expressive speech is absent or virtually so. Under this restriction, only cases of deaf–mutism in which the use of hearing aids or special education has resulted in the development of speech comprehension whilst oral–verbal expression has failed to be acquired, could be taken into account. But such cases seem to be extremely rare. For instance, there are apparently few deaf individuals, if any, who have learned to lip-read but not to speak.

The speech of deaf people may be difficult to understand. Being aware of their limited intelligibility, some individuals may use speech only sparingly, resorting primarily to written or signed language to express themselves. Yet, they can hardly be said to be mute, since they are not totally devoid of speaking abilities.

Developmental Mutism of Central Origin

A number of individuals are born with cerebral lesions or suffer cerebral damage early in life, as a consequence of which they are prevented from acquiring the ability to speak. If these persons acquire verbal comprehension while remaining unable to talk, they are said to have developmental mutism of central origin.

Developmental mutism can be a component of various syndromes.

Cerebral palsy

In some cases, the inability to speak results from cerebral palsy. This is a condition in which the voluntary innervation of the musculature is limited, or perturbed by involuntary muscle contractions. In severe cases, the patients are confined to a wheelchair and are unable to produce intelligible speech or legible script. The inability to utter understandable words is usually concomitant with chewing and swallowing difficulties (dysphagia).

In contradistinction to patients with total functional mutism, cerebral palsied people who cannot speak intelligibly do not usually keep completely silent. They often produce grunts or inarticulate sounds to draw their caretakers' attention or to convey elementary affects.

In some cerebral palsied patients the brain lesions are such that they prevent the acquisition not only of speaking skills but also of age-appropriate speech comprehension. These patients should be considered to have developmental sensory–motor aphasia rather than mutism, because their verbal comprehension remains limited. Only cerebral palsied patients who have adequate verbal competence, i.e. those who have acquired age-appropriate internal command of language but are prevented by motor difficulties from using their linguistic knowledge orally, can truly be said to have mutism. In these people linguistic competence is normal or nearly so but oral–verbal performance is zero.

In a number of cases, it is possible to free the mute patients from their prison of silence by teaching them to use a specially devised typewriter or word processor, or to activate a speech synthesiser. For instance, at the age of 30, Richard Boydell was given a Possum typewriter which he could control with his foot. With this machine he wrote a short autobiographical sketch which was reproduced by Fourcin (1975):

> Like every child, I was born without language. Unfortunately, I was also born with cerebral palsy which, in my case, means that, although my intelligence is unimpaired, I have a very severe speech defect and no use of my hands and arms. So, to start with, I acquired an understanding of language by listening to those around me. Later, thanks to my mother's tireless, patient work I began learning to read and so became familiar with written, as well as with spoken language... When people visited us, either other children or my parents' friends, I enjoyed listening to the conversation even though I could only play a passive role and could not take an active part in any discussion or argument... At the age of 30, I started using the Possum typewriter and, for the first time, had the opportunity to express myself.

Another instance is Christopher Nolan, who uses an electric typewriter the keys of which he activates with a 'unicorn', i.e. a curved stick attached to his forehead. While typing in this way, Nolan needs somebody's help to hold and stabilise his head.

Nolan has a very large vocabulary and a literary talent. So far he has written two books, *Dam-burst of Dreams* (1981) and *Under the Eye of the Clock* (1987), which are largely autobiographical and have brought him fame.

These examples should encourage rehabilitation teams to thoroughly assess the linguistic skills and linguistic potentials of cerebral palsied individuals and, in appropriate cases, to design the technical aids which the patients need to use and expand their verbal knowledge.

At times cerebral palsy affects only the corticobulbar tract, sparing the corticospinal fibres. If the corticobulbar tract is severely damaged the muscles involved in speech are paralysed. As a consequence, expressive speech cannot develop. Writing movements, on the contrary, are possible, because they are effected by means of the corticospinal tract. Patients thus afflicted learn to express themselves in writing.

This form of developmental mutism is sometimes called 'infantile supranuclear mutism' or 'infantile pseudobulbar mutism'. Its symptomatology resembles that of pseudobulbar mutism, which is a form of acquired mutism (see p. 69).

Developmental motor aphasia

A number of individuals are unable to acquire speech although their speech musculature, in contradistinction to that of cerebral palsied patients, is not paralysed and does not evidence involuntary, uncontrollable contractions. These patients may also be unable to learn to whistle or to clear their throat or blow their cheeks on request. Indeed, any deliberate and coordinated activation of the oropharyngeal and laryngeal musculature is impaired.

Although it may not be age appropriate, their comprehension of speech is adequate for everyday interaction. Moreover, the patients can usually acquire some command of written language.

On formal psychometric testing they generally achieve a score a little below norm. Their slight mental handicap may in part be due to their lack of speech, in particular to their inability to ask questions.

This condition can conveniently be referred to as 'developmental motor aphasia'. Some use the name 'congenital motor aphasia' instead. The Germans speak of 'Hörstummheit' (= audio-mutitas) which stresses the fact that the absence of speech is not due to a hearing impairment.

A case of developmental motor aphasia was reported by Lenneberg (1962; 1967, pp. 305–309). His patient was a 4-year-old boy whose verbal comprehension was age appropriate but who could not speak, although his speech musculature was not paralysed. He had no chewing or swallowing difficulties and would spontaneously make sounds when playing and produce grunts when trying to communicate by gestures. Spontaneous laughing and crying had been present since birth and appeared essentially normal. However, he could not perform speech movements. In addition, he found it difficult to produce voice on request. For instance, he was unable to make the pointer of a VU meter of a tape-recorder jump by intentionally coughing into a microphone, although he was aware of the logical connection between sound emission and pointer displacement.

The child was followed up for 4 years. During this period he received speech therapy and learned to repeat a few isolated words with the support of an adult. Therapy failed to teach him to speak. On the other hand, he acquired some command of written language.

This case very much resembles that of a wild child, Victor of Aveyron, described by Itard (1801, 1807) at the beginning of the nineteenth century. Victor had been found roaming in the woods of Lacaune in the south of France. When captured, the boy was wild and speechless. Itard undertook to educate him. Victor learned to understand simple speech and to use a few written words. However, despite intensive training, he could not be taught to speak. He remained mute until his death some 25 years later (Lane, 1977). One of the possible explanations for his persistent mutism is that he had developmental motor aphasia (Lebrun, 1978b, 1980).

Lenneberg was not in favour of calling his case an instance of developmental motor aphasia. He preferred to label his patient's condition 'congenital anarthria' because, he said, 'aphasia' traditionally refers to an acquired disorder resulting from a cortical or subcortical lesion. He felt that in this case the impairment, which was developmental, was probably due to a congenital mesencephalic lesion.

It may be argued, however, that the label 'aphasia' is more appropriate than 'anarthria', because the latter generally implies adequate command of written language (Lebrun, 1989). Moreover, when used without a qualifier it usually refers, like 'aphasia', to an acquired disorder. If it denotes a developmental condition, this generally has to be specified by an adjective such as 'developmental'. Lenneberg used 'congenital' instead, but this can be criticised on the grounds that 'congenital' usually means 'already present at birth'. Although the cause of the speechlessness in Lenneberg's case may conceivably have been present at birth, the speechlessness itself was not (or, if one insists that it was, then it must be conceded that it was not pathological, because no newborn is able to speak).

For these various reasons, the diagnostic label 'congenital anarthria', suggested by Lenneberg, does not appear more appropriate than 'developmental motor aphasia'; indeed the latter seems the more adequate of the two.

It should be mentioned, however, that developmental motor aphasia does not necessarily imply mutism. Some children with this syndrome can produce speech, but their articulation is poor and their active vocabulary generally limited. Only a small number of individuals with developmental motor aphasia have no speech at all. Even in Lenneberg's (1962) patient speech was not totally absent because, after much training, the boy was able to repeat a few words in unison with his speech therapist or his mother.

On the other hand, patients like Richard Boydell, Christopher Nolan, Victor of Aveyron and the boy described by Lenneberg show that it is possible to learn to understand speech although failing to develop concomitant speaking skills. Indeed, a normal verbal competence can be achieved in the absence of intelligible speech, as the case of Boydell and of Nolan demonstrates.

Developmental speech apraxia

In contradistinction to Victor of Aveyron and Lenneberg's patient, some children acquire a good command of written language despite their persistent inability to talk. In a case reported by Elliott and Needleman (1976) the patient, a 6-year-old mute girl, even showed superior reading and writing skills.

Persistent inability to learn to speak in children proficient in the use of written language is usually referred to as 'developmental speech apraxia'. This diagnostic label implies that the child has normal speech comprehension.

An instance of this condition was reported by Smayling (1959). The patient was a 10-year-old boy who was completely mute. Although superiorly intelligent, courteous and outgoing, he could not talk. Indeed, he had never been heard to utter the slightest grunt. His command of written language was age appropriate. On examination, he proved to have poor volitional control of respiratory and palatopharyngeal movements. Intentional lingual and labial displacements lacked specificity, and diadochokinetic rates for articulators were below norm. He could not produce voice on order.

Intensive individual speech therapy was given and the boy's articulatory skills started to develop. However, although he would now use the little speech he had with his mother, he remained silent at school. Probably he was too self-conscious to utter poorly articulated words in front of his classmates. It was not until adequate articulatory skills had been acquired that he could be persuaded to speak and read aloud in the classroom. He was in his sixth year of schooling when he talked for the first time to other pupils.

This case is therefore an instance of developmental speech apraxia evolving into defective speech with selective mutism. Selective mutism could be eliminated by improving speech (see also p. 34).

Acquired Mutism of Central Origin

Contrary to developmental mutism, acquired mutism begins after the individual has acquired speech. Patients with developmental mutism have never been able to speak, whereas patients with acquired mutism had expressive speech before their neurological affection began. Developmental mutism is a failure to acquire speaking skills, whilst acquired mutism is a loss of existing speaking abilities. This loss can be a component of various neurological syndromes

Pseudobulbar palsy

Bilateral lesions affecting the pyramidal tracts in the cerebral hemispheres may bring about a severe condition known as 'pseudobulbar palsy'. Generally, both the corticobulbar and the corticospinal pathways are affected. As a result, the speech muscles are paralysed together with some of the muscles moving the extremities.

Because only the upper motor neurones are injured, the palsied muscles show no wasting and there are no fasciculations. The affected musculature is spastic. Due to hypertonicity, the tongue may appear firmer than normal.

In pseudobulbar palsy, chewing difficulties are frequent and there may be sialorrhoea (constant drooling). If the condition is severe, speech is impossible.

In contrast to the absence of speech movements and of voluntary facial movements, there are unintentional affective contractions of facial muscles, so-called 'spasmodic laughter' and 'spasmodic weeping'. These uncontrollable emotional expressions occur independently of the patient's actual mood. They may be fairly frequent. Also, some spontaneous movements of the lips or of the tongue may occasionally be observed, which the patient cannot reproduce voluntarily.

Prognosis

The prognosis for pseudobulbar mutism is uncertain. At times, spontaneous improvement eventually occurs, absence of speech being replaced by slurred, dysarthric verbal output. As an example a case reported by Bak, Van Dongen and Arts (1983) may be quoted. The patient was a 6-year-old boy who had pseudobulbar palsy of vascular origin. He was totally mute. Neuroradiologically, only one cerebral lesion could be discovered, namely a small infarct in the left thalamus. But neurological symptomatology was bilateral – most probably there was a lesion in both cerebral hemispheres.

Two months after onset, tongue, lip and velum motility had almost completely returned, dysphagia had cleared up and phonation had normalised. Initial mutism had been replaced by dysarthric but intelligible speech.

Unfortunately, in other cases mutism proves more durable. It may even be therapy resistant, as a case reported by Lebrun, Dierick and Hosselaer (1986) shows. Their patient was a Dutch-speaking schoolboy who at age 6;6 years, while he was having a bath, suddenly lost consciousness. He was admitted to the hospital where a spontaneous haemorrhage in the left hemisphere was diagnosed. Craniotomy was performed and an intracerebral blood collection was evacuated. During the first two postoperative weeks, the boy was semi-comatose. When he regained full consciousness, it was observed that his comprehension of simple oral language was moderately impaired whilst oral expression was totally impossible. There was bilateral hyperreflexia and a Babinski sign on either side. The patient had right-sided hemiplegia and hypaesthesia (diminished sensitivity on one side of the body). Movements on the left were possible but slightly ataxic. However, there was no cerebellar syndrome. EEG was diffusely disturbed especially on the left, and the CT scan showed a hypodense zone in the vicinity of the left internal capsule.

The boy was given intensive language and speech therapy. Oral comprehension normalised and the patient learned again to read and write.

However, due to the severe supranuclear paralysis of the speech musculature, he remained completely mute; although he could produce voice on request and sustain phonation for several seconds, he could not articulate a single word. When amused, he would laugh but his laughter was never loud, and retraction of the labial commissures was limited, especially on the right. The boy could not purse his lips, stick out his tongue or puff up his cheeks voluntarily. He had sialorrhoea and could not chew hard food. This condition remained unchanged during the 8 years he was followed up (Lebrun, 1988b).

At times pseudobulbar mutism, a truly organic condition, appears aggravated by psychological factors, as in a case reported by Van Hout (1976) and by Doms (1976). Their patient was a right-handed, moderately alcoholic male who, at the age of 31, had a severe car accident, in which his passenger was killed. He himself suffered a severe head trauma which caused immediate coma. The patient was admitted to the hospital. Due to respiratory problems, he had to undergo tracheotomy and be artificially ventilated. A left carotid arteriogram indicated some oedema in the temporal lobe and deviation of the anterior cerebral artery to the right. The patient was unconscious. He had quadriparesis and on noxious stimulation showed bilateral decerebration movements.

This condition persisted for about 3 months. During this period he had several urinary infections and aspiration pneumonia with secondary atelectasis. He also developed a sacral bedsore. Eventually consciousness started to return. Spontaneous movements could be observed on the left. Respiration was now normal again and the tracheostoma could be closed. Swallowing was still difficult. The patient often choked on liquids or regurgitated them. Moreover, he was unable to speak. Only from time to time could he produce an isolated sound or syllable, uttered in a faint voice. Ten months after the accident, neurological examination showed the patient to have right-sided hemiplegia with ankylosis of the elbow in flexion. There was some spasticity on the left with reduced mobility. Swallowing was now nearly normal but the patient was still completely mute. Physical, occupational and speech therapies were given but did not seem to be well accepted. In point of fact, the patient appeared disinterested and often kept aloof.

Five years after the cerebral trauma, mutism was still complete. However, the patient had no aphasia and no oral apraxia. He expressed himself by means of an alphabetical board, pointing in quick succession to the letters forming the words he wanted to use. Due to his right hemiplegia and severe retropulsion he could not leave his wheelchair. He had a right inferior facial paralysis. Voluntary lingual movements were slow, particularly to the right. The tongue could be protruded and was not deviated. When the patient attempted to phonate his velum remained practically immobile on the right whilst it moved slightly on the left. The left vocal cord was found to be paretic. During attempts to phonate, closure of the vocal chink remained incomplete. There was reduced ventilation with limited diaphragmatic excursion, particularly on the right. The patient was audible when coughing or laughing. He could voluntarily phonate for a very short period of time but could not speak. Only isolated sounds or short syllables could be produced after much stimulation and in a faint voice. Very occasionally a polysyllabic word could be elicited, but the patient had to pause after each syllable.

Although this man undoubtedly had very severe motor deficits, there may be some question as to whether his persistent mutism was entirely organic. Since only his velum was paralysed bilaterally, he should have been able to produce at least short sentences. Most probably, his verbal output would have been strongly nasalised, and moreover, due to the paresis of the left vocal cord, his voice would have sounded breathy. But there should have been some speech. Why then did the patient remain mute? Maybe, when he regained consciousness, he was so severely handicapped that he really could not speak at all; in fact, he had difficulty even in swallowing. But he may have soon discovered that he could derive benefit from his speechlessness. Being mute he could not be expected to vindicate his behaviour and to answer the reproaches of his parents who considered him responsible for the car accident which he had had and which had killed his passenger. Moreover, although she was reproachful of his conduct, the patient's mother became overprotective to her handicapped son. The patient's wife also tended to approach him maternally, as if he were an infant. In addition, she taught him to use an alphabetical board. Accordingly, the patient could express his most urgent needs without having to use speech. These various factors may have contributed to the fixation of the muteness and may explain why the patient did not really accept the speech therapy he was given and why he did not respond to the suggestion which was made to teach him to use a typewriter.

If speech therapy had been started as soon as the patient regained consciousness and if, in addition to providing services to the patient, the therapist had been able to influence the behaviour of his relatives, the expressive skills might possibly have been improved, thus preventing mutism from becoming irreversible.

In patients with pseudobulbar palsy the paralysis affecting the extremities at times resolves, whilst the speech musculature remains paralysed and speech impossible. As an example the third case reported by Grosswasser *et al.* (1988) may be quoted. Their patient was a young, hypertensive woman. At the age of 25, she suffered a first stroke which entailed transient right hemiparesis and dysphagia. Six years later, she had a second stroke which resulted in left hemiparesis and inability to speak. In addition, the patient was unable to perform orofacial movements voluntarily and she had swallowing difficulties. There was no aphasia, and the patient expressed herself in writing.

The hemiparesis cleared within 6 weeks but paralysis of the speech musculature and mutism remained. They were still present 3 years after onset.

Improvement or even normalisation of movements in the extremities is therefore no guarantee that mutism can be conquered.

Opercular syndrome

The speech musculature may also show flaccid paralysis in the absence of significant impairment of movements in the extremities. This affection is called 'the opercular syndrome'. Other names are 'flaccid facial diplegia', 'facio-labio-linguopharyngeal palsy of cortico-subcortical origin', and 'Foix–Chavany–Marie syndrome'.

The main clinical feature of the opercular syndrome is a very severe reduction of the voluntary motility of oral, pharyngeal, and at times also laryngeal, muscles. The lips, tongue and mandible can barely be moved deliberately. As a consequence, mastication is hampered, as is the first stage of swallowing, and speech is precluded. The soft palate does not move on attempts to phonate. At rest, the mouth tends to be half open and the face generally looks void. However, there is no muscle wasting and no fasciculation because only the upper motor neurones are affected.

At times the paralysis extends to the upper facial musculature. The patient is unable to close his eyes or to frown voluntarily. Facial diplegia is then complete.

Whereas volitional innervation of the facio-labiopharyngeal musculature is severely limited, automatic movements are present. Normal mimic reactions are observed when the patient is amused or emotionally moved, and the second phase of swallowing, which is reflexive in nature, is usually undisturbed. Reflex cough and spontaneous yawning are also present.

If the upper facial musculature is affected, the patient cannot close his eyelids, move his eyeballs or frown on command, but he does so reflexly.

There is therefore a striking automatic–voluntary dissociation in the opercular syndrome: intentional innervation is impaired whereas reflex and spontaneous emotional innervations are preserved.

Whilst their affective facial expressions tend to be normal, patients with the opercular syndrome do not as a rule show the excessive emotionality which is often observed in patients with pseudobulbar palsy.

The opercular syndrome usually results from damage to the two opercula Rolandi and their efferent fibres. In each cerebral hemisphere the operculum Rolandi (also called the 'operculum frontoparietalis') is the lower part of the pre- and postcentral convolutions (Figure 3).

Because both opercula Rolandi are damaged, some authors refer to the disease as the 'bi-opercular syndrome'.

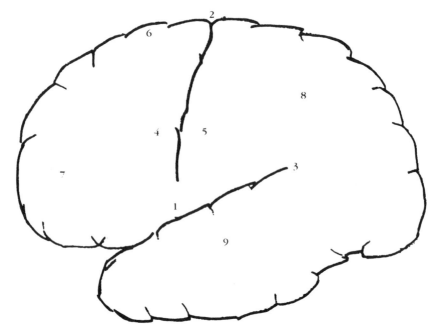

Figure 3. Sketch of the lateral aspect of the left cerebral hemisphere: (1) operculum Rolandi or frontoparietal operculum; (2) central sulcus or fissure of Rolando; (3) lateral sulcus or sylvian fissure; (4) precentral gyrus; (5) postcentral gyrus; (6) supplementary motor area; (7) frontal lobe; (8) parietal lobe; (9) temporal lobe.

Anamnestically it is often found that the patient first suffered a cerebrovascular accident in one hemisphere, which entailed transient motor difficulties, including motor speech problems. Later, he suffered a stroke in the other hemisphere, as a result of which the opercular syndrome emerged.

The first instance of the opercular syndrome reported in the medical literature seems to be the case published in 1837 by Magnus and summarised by Alajouanine and Thurel in 1933. The patient was a 25-year-old female who suffered a double cerebrovascular accident as a result of which she lost her faculty of speech. In addition to being unable to speak, the patient could not contract facial muscles voluntarily, but did so reflexly. Chewing was extremely difficult, whereas deglutition was easy. The patient had to use her finger to push food to the back of the mouth cavity from where it could be swallowed. Spontaneous laughing was entirely normal. Voluntary phonation was possible, but could not be accompanied by articulatory movements. The facial musculature was hypotonic and at rest the face was expressionless.

Alajouanine and Thurel (1933) themselves reported the case of a 41-year-old male who had suddenly become mute and had at first been diagnosed as having hysterical mutism. The voluntary motility of the labio-glossopharyngeal musculature was severely reduced. The patient could not chew. He could only drink fluids, which he had to pour in his mouth with his head tilted backwards. This manoeuvre was not always successful, however, and the patient often choked on liquids. He died of aspiration pneumonia some time later.

Another typical example was reported by Cappa *et al.* (1987). The patient was a 50-year-old woman with insulin-dependent diabetes. She suffered at first a stroke in the left hemisphere which caused transient right-sided hemiparesis and dysarthria. Three months later she suffered a stroke in the right hemisphere which rendered her completely mute and entailed swallowing difficulties. Voluntary contractions of the facial, labial and lingual musculature was either impossible or extremely limited. At rest, the face looked void. Spontaneous laughing and weeping were preserved, but appeared a little stereotyped. Voice could be produced on request. Examination disclosed no aphasia and no apraxia. The patient had no comprehension difficulty and expressed herself correctly and fluently in writing. The CT scan documented a bilateral vascular lesion. On the left, the lesion appeared limited to the operculum Rolandi. On the right it was larger and involved the operculum Rolandi together with some adjacent areas.

The opercular syndrome may also occur in children. For instance, Chateau *et al.* (1966) described a child who suffered from acute meningoencephalitis shortly after he had started to speak. The disease rendered him mute. When seen aged 7 years, the boy could not voluntarily contract his facio-labiopharyngeal musculature. He could not speak and had severe dysphagia. However, his spontaneous affective facial expressions were vivid and stood in sharp contrast to his facial atony at rest.

The patient had been given speech therapy, but to no avail. He could not use his speech musculature volitionally. Therefore, it was decided to teach him to write. Acquisition of written language proved possible and the patient learned to express himself in writing.

Mutism associated with a pyramidal hemisyndrome

Mutism can be accompanied by hemiplegia involving the face as well as the extremities on the same side. In other words, loss of speech may be associated with a pyramidal hemisyndrome.

Such a case was reported by Jude and Trabaud in 1928. Their patient, a 24-year-old soldier, had mutism with left hemiplegia and facial palsy on the same side, without sensory deficits. The paralysis was more pronounced in the upper than in the lower limb. There were some chewing and swallowing difficulties. The patient had no oral comprehension disorder and could read and write normally. But he could not utter a single word. His complete silence was interrupted from time to time by an uncontrollable fit of uproarious laughter which occurred independently of the situation and of his actual mood.

Alajouanine *et al.* (1959b) reported the case of a right-handed man who suddenly developed mutism with right facial paralysis and right-sided hemiplegia without loss of sensitivity. As in the preceding case, the upper limb was more affected than the lower limb. The patient could not contract his facio-labiolingual musculature at will, except for his masseters. He had only slight dysphagia and his affective facial expressions were normal.

The patient was totally unable to speak. He had no comprehension difficulty and expressed himself in writing. He wrote correctly but slowly on account of his having to use his left hand.

Arteriography disclosed a subcortical infarction involving the lenticular nucleus, the caudate nucleus and the internal capsule on the left. Right-sided carotid arteriography was normal.

A somewhat comparable case was reported by Chia and Kinsbourne (1987). Their patient was a right-handed Chinese who had mutism and right spastic hemiplegia following what appears in CT scans to be a bleeding involving the left basal ganglia. This man expressed himself in writing, using his non-preferred hand. However, he wrote mirror-wise, reversing each individual ideogram along its vertical axis. He ordered the columns of writing from right to left, however, as is normal in written Chinese. When requested to produce correctly oriented ideograms, he found it difficult to comply with the instruction.

At times extremities are only paretic. Indeed, there may be motor neglect rather than paralysis, as a case reported by Berthier, Starkstein and Leiguarda (1987) and by Starkstein, Berthier and Leiguarda (1988) shows. Their patient was a 55-year-old right-handed male who suddenly presented with mutism, left lower facial paralysis, severe dysphagia and inability to contract his labial and lingual musculature voluntarily. Spontaneous coughing and yawning were present. The patient did not move his left limbs either spontaneously or in reaction to painful stimuli. However, when urged to look at his left extremities and to move them, he could do so, demonstrating only mild hemiparesis.

A case briefly described by Damasio *et al.* (1982) seems to belong to the same group. The patient was an 82-year-old man who became suddenly mute with left hemiparesis. He had no aphasia but showed left unilateral neglect.

Neuropathology

In the cases of Alajouanine *et al.* (1959b) and of Chia and Kinsbourne (1987) the lesion was in the left hemisphere. In the cases reported by Mendel (1912, 1914), Jude and Trabaud (1928), Souques (1928), Damasio *et al.* (1982), and Starkstein, Berthier and Leiguarda (1988), on the contrary, it was in the right hemisphere. A patient may then be rendered mute by a unilateral lesion in the left or right hemisphere, independent of his manual preference (the patients of Alajouanine *et al.* and of Chia and Kinsbourne were right handed just as the patients of Mendel, Damasio *et al.* and Starkstein, Berthier and Leiguarda).

Maybe Pierre Marie (1906a,b) was thinking of this when he claimed that 'anarthria', i.e. the selective loss of oral–verbal expression, could result from a lesion in the left as well as from a lesion in the right hemisphere.

In the cases of Alajouanine *et al.*, Damasio *et al.* and Chia and Kinsbourne neuroradiology disclosed a subcortical lesion. In the cases of Mendel and Starkstein, Berthier and Leiguarda, the lesion was at autopsy found to be cortico-subcortical. In Mendel's case, it involved the grey and white matter of the third frontal and first temporal convolutions as well as of the insula. In the case of Starkstein, Berthier and Leiguarda, it involved the insula, the inner surface of the operculum and part of the corona radiata. (In the cases reported by Jude and Trabaud, and by Souques, the exact site of the lesion in the right hemisphere could not be assessed.)

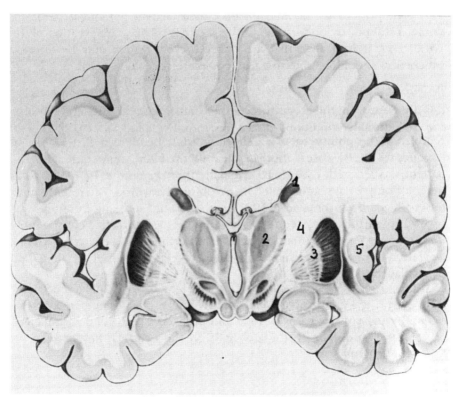

Figure 4. Coronal section through the cerebral hemispheres and the brainstem: (1) caudate nucleus; (2) thalamus; (3) lenticular nucleus; (4) internal capsule; (5) insula.

Mutism with hemiplegia may therefore result from a cortico-subcortical or a pure subcortical lesion in the area which Marie (1906a) called 'the lenticular zone'. Head (1926, p.70) referred to this area as 'Pierre Marie's quadrilateral'. It extends from the convolutions of the insula to the lenticular nucleus and its adjacent structures, probably including the internal capsule (Figure 4).

The case described by Petit-Dutaillis et al. in 1954 differs in several respects from those discussed above. The patient had right-sided hemiplegia but no significant facial weakness. His lower limb was more affected than his upper limb. He had no dysphagia and could freely move his tongue and lips. The causal lesion was a bleeding aneurysm on one of the branches of the anterior cerebral artery in the posterior part of the first left frontal convolution. This zone is often called 'Penfield's supplementary motor area' (see Figures 3 and 5).

In this case of mutism accompanied by a pyramidal hemisyndrome sparing the face, surgical resection of the aneurysm resulted in the return of speech and the gradual improvement of the hemiplegia.

Pathophysiology

The pathophysiology of mutism associated with a pyramidal hemisyndome is still poorly understood. In view of the bilateral innervation of the vocal tract, it is strange that a unilateral lesion which may be entirely subcortical should be able to cause complete speech suspension.

Prognosis

It is not clear from the literature whether mutism due to a unilateral lesion can be a durable condition. After a few months, Mendel's (1912) patient recovered the ability to utter short words. She died a little later. In Souques's (1928) cases, mutism cleared up after some time and the patient was left with dysarthria. The patient of Damasio et al. (1982) was mute for only 2 days, after which he exhibited dysarthria. Ten months after onset Chia and Kinsbourne's (1987) patient could speak again but he was severely dysarthric. Fourteen months later, his dysarthria had considerably improved. As for the patient of Starkstein, Berthier and Leiguarda (1988), he started to utter isolated speech sounds 1 week after onset. He then died of cardiac arrest.

These observations suggest that mutism caused by a unilateral lesion tends to be less permanent than mutism due to pseudobulbar or to bi-opercular palsy. (The cases of Jude and Trabaud (1928) and Alajouanine et al. (1959b) do not throw any light on the issue as they contain no follow-up information.)

Differential diagnosis

Clinicians do not always clearly distinguish between pseudobulbar palsy, the opercular syndrome and a pyramidal hemisyndrome and yet, a number of features generally make a distinction possible. For instance, in pseudobulbar paralysis the affected musculature is spastic, whereas in the opercular syndrome it is hypotonic. In the former disease, paralysis of the speech musculature is often accompanied by a motor deficit in one or more extremities, whilst this is rarely the case in the opercular syndrome. Finally, in pseudobulbar palsy, spasmodic laughter and spasmodic weeping are frequent whereas they are not observed in the opercular syndrome.

On the other hand, in cases of mutism accompanied by a pyramidal hemisyndrome facial paralysis is unilateral or absent, whereas it is bilateral in pseudobulbar palsy and in the opercular syndrome. Moreover, in the latter two affections there is a striking automatic–voluntary dissociation which is not observed in cases of mutism with a pyramidal hemisyndrome.

Although it is generally possible to distinguish between the three conditions, there are undoubtedly borderline cases where a diagnostic decision is difficult, if not impossible. For instance, there may be some dispute as to whether the case reported both by Berthier, Starkstein and Leiguarda (1987) and by Starkstein, Berthier and Leiguarda (1988) should not be regarded as an instance of the opercular syndrome rather than as an instance of mutism associated with a pyramidal hemisyndrome. In point of fact, Starkstein, Berthier and Leiguarda (1988) considered that their clinical findings 'suggest(ed) the opercular syndrome'. It is a fact that their patient's pyramidal hemisyndrome was slight in the extremities. He had hemiparesis whilst patients suffering from mutism associated with a pyramidal hemisyndrome generally have hemiplegia. However, the patient of Starkstein, Berthier and Leiguarda had unilateral facial paralysis instead of the facial diplegia which is typical of the opercular syndrome and, in addition, he had a unilateral lesion and this lesion completely spared the external surface of the operculum Rolandi. Admittedly a number of patients have been reported who had an opercular lesion on one side only (see Alajouanine et al., 1953a; Boudin, Pepin and Wiart, 1960; Pertuiset and Perrier, 1960), but these patients, although they had dysarthria, were not mute.

For these various reasons, it would seem that the case reported by Berthier's team is to be regarded as an instance of mutism accompanied by a pyramidal hemisyndrome rather than as the first reported case 'of a bilateral opercular syndrome due to a right-hemispheric lesion' (Starkstein, Berthier and Leiguarda, 1988).

This example shows that, by virtue of their nature, extent, and location, cerebral lesions may at times bring about complex conditions which cannot be easily classified. However, the existence of atypical or mixed cases should not deter the accurate diagnosis of patients whenever possible.

Oral apraxia

Some authors construe the inability of pseudobulbar or opercular syndrome patients to perform voluntary facio-oropharyngeal movements as oral apraxia. This does not seem to be an adequate interpretation. It is a fact that in these patients a dissociation can often be observed between intentional and unintentional innervation of the facio-labio-glossopharyngeal musculature. Yet, the inability to voluntarily innervate this musculature does not seem to be apraxic in nature. By definition, apraxia is a disorder of learned gestures. Therefore, oral apraxia typically spares chewing and swallowing movements, which are movements nobody needs to learn. In other words, oral apraxia does not cause dysphagia or sialorrhoea. But patients with pseudobulbar palsy or the opercular syndrome do have chewing and swallowing difficulties and may have constant drooling.

Moreover, apraxia is typically observed in the absence of significant paralysis. Apraxics, except sometimes immediately after onset, do make movements, but not the appropriate ones. Apraxia does not impair motility as such, but hampers the organisation of learned purposive movements. In patients with pseudobulbar palsy or with the opercular syndrome, on the contrary, voluntary innervation of the musculature is precluded. The muscles are paralysed as far as volitional movements are concerned.

Finally, it may be reasoned that if the facio-labio-glossopharyngeal deficit in pseudobulbar palsy and the opercular syndrome were apraxic in nature, it would, like most apraxic syndromes (with the notable exception of apraxia for dressing), be precipitated far more frequently by a lesion in the left than by a lesion in the right hemisphere. This, however, is not the case. Whilst voluntary innervation of the said musculature generally breaks down after the patient has incurred a second (sometimes a third or fourth) cerebral lesion, the triggering lesion may be located in the left or in the right hemisphere. It suffices that it is not on the same side as the preceding injuries.

For these various reasons, it appears inappropriate to classify the inability of patients with pseudobulbar palsy or the opercular syndrome to contract their facio-glossopharyngeal musculature at will as oral apraxia.

Terminology

Selective loss of expressive speech, i.e. loss of oral–verbal expression with preservation of all other verbal abilities, has been variously referred to in the literature. Some authors, including Petit-Dutaillis *et al.* (1964), Alajouanine *et al.* (1959b) and Starkstein, Berthier and Leiguarda (1988) used the term 'aphemia', which was originally introduced by Paul Broca (1861) to denote selective loss of articulate speech in the absence of paralysis of the oropharyngeal musculature. Others, including Jude and

Trabaud (1928) and Souques (1928), used the term 'anarthria', which was vindicated by Pierre Marie (1906a,b). Still others, especially in the early years of the twentieth century, spoke of 'motor aphasia'. This is what Mendel (1912, 1914) did in connection with his case of selective speechlessness. Other aphasiologists used the term 'pure motor aphasia' or 'subcortical motor aphasia' to refer to the isolated loss of expressive speech. They contrasted this condition with 'Broca's aphasia' or 'cortical motor aphasia' which, in addition to non-existent or sparse oral–verbal output, included agraphia and alexia.

Affections of the motor neurones

Pseudobulbar mutism, opercular mutism and mutism associated with a pyramidal hemisyndrome are usually caused by one or several lesions which are vascular or traumatic in nature. These lesions injure upper motor neurones, causing paralysis.

Motor neurones may also be affected by diseases of the central nervous system. Degeneration of the motor neurones results in impaired motility. When the innervation of the speech muscles is severely compromised, the patients can no longer speak. This type of acquired mutism may be a component of several maladies.

Motor neurone disease

Motor neurone disease, also called 'amyotrophic lateral sclerosis' (ALS), is a degenerative affection of the corticobulbar and corticospinal tracts, the bulbar motor nuclei and the anterior horns of the medulla. Generally both the upper and lower motor neurones are affected but to a variable degree.

If the upper motor neurones are primarily impaired, the symptomatology is reminiscent of pseudobulbar palsy. For instance, in a case reported by Lieberman and Benson (1977), mutism was accompanied by excessive emotional expression. The patient was aware of her exaggerated affective display and vainly tried to control it.

Having lost the ability to speak, she expressed herself in writing. As her motor neurone disease progressed, she also lost the ability to write. In order to communicate, she then used the Morse code which she implemented by means of eyelid movements.

If the disease affects primarily the lower motor neurones, the symptomatology resembles what is observed in bulbar palsy.

Bulbar palsy

Bulbar palsy is an impairment of the lower motor neurones, specifically of the nuclei of the cranial nerves in the bulb. It causes flaccid paralysis of the speech musculature with muscle wasting and fasciculations. In severe cases, the speech muscles can no longer contract and no audible speech can be produced.

Bulbar mutism is usually accompanied by severe dysphagia. In a number of cases, the swallowing difficulties result in the inhalation of food, and this may cause the patient's death.

Multiple sclerosis

Multiple sclerosis is an affection of the white matter which becomes demyelinated at various places scattered throughout the central nervous system. The areas of demyelination, called 'plaques', interfere with the transmission of nerve impulses. The interference may be severe and prevent the speech muscles from being innervated. The patient is then unable to produce speech. If he is also unable to write, his condition, from the point of view of communication, resembles that of cerebral palsied patients (see p. 65).

Multiple sclerosis patients who can no longer produce intelligible speech or script can usually be taught to use a speech synthesiser, a special typewriter or a word processor to express themselves.

In some cases, the severity of the symptoms varies with time. There are periods of exacerbation and of partial remission. In other cases, the course of the disease is slowly but irreversibly progressive.

Hepatolenticular degeneration

Hepatolenticular degeneration, also called 'Wilson's disease', is a disturbance of copper metabolism. Deposits of the metal form in various parts of the body including the brain. If left untreated, the illness generally brings about a neuromotor degeneration which may eventually result in mutism.

Myasthenia gravis

Myasthenia gravis is an affection of the myoneural junction. Clinically, patients suffering from this disease show progressive weakness with repeated use, and recovery with rest. If the speech musculature is affected, the patients, after they have been talking for some time, experience increasing difficulty in producing audible speech, until they become completely mute. After a period of rest, they can resume speaking, but if they keep talking, muscle fatigue gradually reappears and temporary mutism eventually ensues.

Patients who are rendered mute as a consequence of myasthenia gravis differ from patients who are mute as a result of motor neurone disease or bulbar palsy in that their mutism, although recurrent, is not permanent. After each period of rest, they can speak again, albeit transiently.

The condition of patients with myasthenia gravis can usually be improved with drugs, e.g. neostigmine (Prostigmine).

Therapy

Clinicians are generally agreed that when mutism caused by a progressive affection of the neuromotor system cannot be improved by drugs, very little can be done to help the patient regain some oral–verbal abilities. In order to be of some benefit to the patient, speech therapy must be initiated before mutism sets in, preferably as soon as the first signs of dysarthria are detected. If started early enough, speech therapy can help slow down motor speech disintegration.

This conservative speech therapy usually aims at teaching the dysarthric patient to constantly monitor his speech performance. Speaking should become a highly conscious, deliberate task. The goals of being heard and understood should replace the former goals of being quick and colourfully expressive. In many cases this can be best achieved by slowing down the speed of delivery, by avoiding reducing unstressed syllables, and by refraining from using words which experience has shown to be particularly difficult to manage.

Simultaneously, the patient should be encouraged to engage in oral–verbal activities. Speech abstinence can only increase the speech production difficulties.

If oral motility is already severely impaired when therapy is started, having the patient practise some simple labial, lingual or velar movements may prove useful.

In addition to providing speech therapy for the patient, it is often desirable to give the relatives some guidance. The entourage should learn to facilitate self-expression by the patient. For instance, they should endeavour to have the patient live in a quiet atmosphere where he does not need to speak overloud to be understood. They should also be instructed not to speak at the same time as the patient and not to interrupt him. They should make it a habit to come close to him when he is speaking, and they should learn not to lose patience if he cannot be readily understood.

Aphasic mutism

Frequently in the neurological literature the word 'mutism' is used to refer to an absence of expressive speech associated with aphasic symptoms. The patient has no oral–verbal output (see Figure 2, p. 59) but, in addition, appears on examination to have some comprehension difficulties and to make linguistic errors when expressing himself in writing.

Although such a condition is in fact a form of motor aphasia, the term 'mutism' is used because the total absence of expressive speech stands in contrast to the relative preservation (or recovery) of speech comprehension.

A case of this nature was reported by David and Bone (1984). Their patient was a 51-year-old right-handed housewife who, following a stroke in the left hemisphere, lost the ability to express herself orally. She had no oral apraxia but was unable to speak, whisper or mouth words either on request or in imitation. Nor could she hum. By contrast, speech comprehension, reading and writing were but mildly impaired. She had no dysphagia. There was a slight central facial weakness on the right.

The absence of oral–verbal output lasted for about 2 months. Then speech returned but it was non-fluent and laboured, and it contained phonemic paraphasias.

A rather similar condition was observed by de Morsier (1949), except that his patient had a slight right-sided hemiparesis together with severe dysphagia and inability to move the tongue. The palatal and gag reflexes were absent. The total speechlessness contrasted strongly with the mild impairment of writing and the absence of comprehension difficulties.

Dysphagia cleared in less than a month. Some time later, speech started to return but, as in David and Bone's (1984) case, it was non-fluent.

In a case reported by Masdeu, Schoene and Funkenstein (1978) articulation was recovered before phonation. After the recovery of voice production, verbal output for some time remained sparse, with occasional phonemic and verbal paraphasias.

In these three cases, aphasic mutism, i.e. mutism occurring in the context of aphasia, was caused by a cerebrovascular accident. In 1976, Lebrun reported a case where aphasic mutism was observed after surgery. The patient was an ambidextrous woman who at 54 years of age started to suffer from jacksonian convulsions with clonic movements of the right eyelid, jaw jerking, pharyngeal stricture, slight respiratory difficulty and inability to speak. Neuroradiology disclosed a tumour in the left hemisphere and the patient was operated upon. A meningioma which pressed on the left operculum Rolandi was excised.

Postoperatively the patient had right-sided facial paralysis with hypaesthesia. When protruded the tongue deviated to the right. Its motility was considerably reduced. The palatal and pharyngeal reflexes were present. Nevertheless, swallowing was difficult. The patient was unable to speak. She would express herself in writing. She wrote slowly because her right hand was paretic. Moreover, she made a number of spelling errors. Comprehension of ordinary speech was preserved but there was some degree of acalculia. Mutism lasted a few weeks. Then speech started to return but it was severely dysarthric. At the same time, the agraphia and acalculia cleared. Dysarthria, though less severe, was still present 2 years after surgery. On the other hand, no sign of aphasia could be detected.

A somewhat similar case was reported by Ruff and Arbit (1981).

Following drainage of a spontaneous haematoma centred in the left middle frontal gyrus and dissected into the white matter of the left inferior frontal and precentral gyri, a 15-year-old right-handed female was unable to produce audible speech. However, she could mouth words soundlessly so that it was sometimes possible to understand her by reading her lips. She could hum the tunes of popular songs correctly and move her tongue and lips freely. She had no dysphagia. What she could not do was to combine expiration and phonation with articulation.

The patient was able to write but made some spelling errors. Use of the pen was poor on account of moderate right-sided motor weakness. Speech comprehension and reading were normal. Three weeks later, the patient started to speak audibly. Her speech was laborious with 'transient word blocking and phonetic disintegration'. Repetition was better than spontaneous speech. In the ensuing months, writing fully normalised and oral–verbal delivery improved.

In these five cases of aphasic mutism speechlessness was eventually conquered, but delivery remained impaired for an appreciable length of time.

Aphasic mutism is not rare after cerebral trauma, especially if the trauma has initially rendered the victim comatose. After the patient regains consciousness, it may be found that comprehension of simple speech is returning whilst expressive speech is still totally absent. For instance, a 12-year-old girl who had sustained closed head injury with ensuing coma, started to obey verbal commands 8 days after the accident. She did not start to speak until 2 weeks later (Levin *et al.*, 1985).

When expressive speech begins to re-emerge, the patient may whisper instead of producing voiced speech. When finally voice re-appears, it may be hoarse.

Before (whispered) speech returns, some patients start giving written responses. Written expression may be recovered before oral expression.

As an instance of such gradual recovery of expressive abilities the case reported by De Mol and Deleval (1979) may be quoted. Their patient was a 9-year-old boy who had been knocked over by a car. He was comatose when admitted to the hospital. When he awoke, he did not speak at all. However, he would occasionally answer questions in writing. This situation lasted for about 2 weeks, when speech started to return. Articulation was correct, but it was aphonic. A few days later, whispering was replaced by voiced speech.

It is still unknown why in some cases of organic mutism control over the articulators is recovered before control over the larynx.

Interestingly, patients in the whispering stage may sometimes be heard to produce voice in reaction to pain or under the influence of an affect. In such cases it is clearly the voluntary innervation of the larynx which is still impaired.

The return of (whispered) speech does not necessarily mean the return of loquacity. Although being able to speak again, the patient may at first remain very taciturn, briefly answering questions but not initiating speech. For instance, Levin (1981, p. 454) mentioned a 2.5-year-old girl with precocious verbal skills. She was involved in a car accident and sustained closed head injury. She was comatose and had right-sided hemiparesis. Some time after she had regained consciousness she started to follow verbal instructions but did not begin to speak until 10 days later. She would give short answers to questions and join in singing but she failed to initiate speech. This taciturnity disappeared gradually.

The absence of (spontaneous) speech in children who have suffered cerebral trauma has impressed many clinicians, who tend to regard it as a hallmark of traumatic aphasia in children.

The syndrome of the Sleeping Beauty

Todorow (1978) has upheld the view that in children the absence of verbal behaviour, and particularly of expressive speech, after sudden brain damage and ensuing coma, is not truly organic in origin: the lack of verbal output and of reactions to verbal stimulation is psychologically based.

According to Todorow, the child who has suffered brain trauma followed by coma and who, on regaining consciousness, finds himself in a totally unknown environment (the hospital), is seized with an overwhelming fear that brings about a psychotic withdrawal characterised by akinesia (lack of movements), abulia (lack of initiative), apathy and mutism. This reactive condition has been called the 'syndrome of the Sleeping Beauty' by Todorow.

However, the reality of this syndrome is debatable. There is no convincing evidence that the absence of verbal behaviour, and particularly of expressive speech, after coma is a psychological reaction elicited by the cerebral aggression which the child has experienced, and by the unfamiliar and weird environment he finds himself in. Rather, the gradual recovery of communicative skills, together with the residual verbal deficits which may persist for years (Levin, 1981; Levin et al., 1983; Lebrun, 1988a) strongly suggests that mutism is organically based.

Todorow's theory is further weakened by the fact that mutism may be observed even when the cerebral trauma does not entail loss of consciousness and, the patient makes visible efforts to speak. For instance, Guttman (1942) described a 6-year-old boy who was admitted to the hospital because he had bumped his head into a lamp-post when riding his bicycle. Although he had a compound fracture of the left frontoparietal region, the child had not lost consciousness. He was operated upon. Bone splinters were removed and his brain wound was toileted. Two days later, he was fully alert. He had right faciobrachial monoplegia. He carried out simple verbal orders, but could not answer questions. He made attempts at speaking, moving his tongue and lips, but could not get a sound out. Four days later, he started to repeat words and to count from one to ten, but he was severely dysarthric. Moreover, he did not answer questions other than by head movements, and he could not name objects held up to him. A few days later, spontaneous speech started to re-emerge. His pronunciation was slurred and difficult to understand. This improved over the next few months, until his articulation was fully normalised.

In such a case, it can hardly be contended that the boy awoke in a weird environment, because he did not lose consciousness, or that he took refuge in mutism and apathy, because he visibly attempted to speak. Moreover, when he started to talk again, he proved to be severely dysarthric, and this dysarthria testifies to the organic origin of his speechlessness.

It should finally be noted that not only children but also adults may be mute after cerebral trauma, and this mutism may last for quite some time.

For instance, Levin *et al.* (1983) observed a 35-year-old factory worker who was comatose following closed head injury. One month after the accident, he opened his eyes. But he did not follow verbal instructions until 6 months later. One year after injury, he demonstrated comprehension of simple spoken and written language and ability to perform simple calculations. However, he was still completely mute and remained so for another 4 months.

In this case, therefore, expressive speech re-emerged 9 months after comprehension of simple speech. There is no reason to suppose that this long-lasting mutism was due to the so-called syndrome of the Sleeping Beauty.

Pathophysiology

Although there is little reason to consider that mutism following brain trauma is reactive, i.e. psychological, in nature, the exact pathophysiology of it is still largely unknown. It may be an extreme form of motor aphasia or it may be due to a severe impairment of speech movements. It may also be a combination of the two disorders. The pathogenesis may actually vary from case to case.

Therapy

Clinicians are generally agreed that it is difficult to tackle post-traumatic mutism directly, because its pathophysiology is not clear. They feel, however, that the patient should be given intensive verbal stimulation and be constantly encouraged to react verbally. This, it is thought, is likely to speed up the return of expressive speech. Once the patient starts to speak again, the therapy should be tailored to the presenting difficulties.

Improper labelling

Whilst it may be legitimate to speak of mutism in cases where the absence of expressive speech stands in contrast to the relatively well preserved (or recovered) comprehension of speech, there seems to be little reason to call mutism the absence or quasi-absence of oral–verbal expression in global aphasia, because by definition patients with global aphasia also have marked comprehension difficulties.

It appears equally inappropriate to speak of mutism in cases of aphasia with recurrent utterance. In fact, patients with this type of aphasia often fail to communicate any better than mute patients. But they are not silent. Indeed, their verbal output, although stereotyped, may be copious. Moreover, these patients often have impaired comprehension of speech and they are generally alexic and agraphic (Lebrun, 1986).

Locked-in syndrome

The locked-in syndrome is a neurological affection in which voluntary motility has broken down completely, but for a few isolated movements, such as vertical eye movements. Some involuntary movements such as sighing, coughing or moaning may occur. In some cases weeping and screaming are observed. Spontaneous laughing, although limited in scope, may be present.

Patients with the locked-in syndrome have spastic quadriplegia. In addition, they are mute but alert. Usually, they have preserved comprehension of simple spoken language and, indeed, their linguistic knowledge may be largely intact. Accordingly, it is sometimes possible to communicate with them by using a code based on one of the few voluntary movements they can still perform. For instance, a patient of Vallar and Cappa (1987) was unable to speak, to write and to make any deliberate movement with the exception of the vertical displacement of the eyeballs, the closure of the eyes and a slight movement of the head. He communicated with those around him by means of eye movements (upward gaze for 'no' and downward gaze for 'yes'), which enabled him to answer yes–no questions and to make a choice in a series of alternatives proposed by the speech partner. He could also use his residual head movement to act on a transducer which was connected with a letter board and a special typewriter. In this way, he could form short written messages. However, he did not resort spontaneously to this means of communication and had to be constantly exhorted, if he was to produce a written answer (Cappa, Prirovano and Vignolo, 1985).

In a case reported by Gauger (1980) the patient could activate a buzzer with his forehead and in this way generate Morse words and sentences.

Pathogenesis

The locked-in syndrome generally results from a lesion severing the pyramidal tract bilaterally in the ventral pons or, less frequently, in the two cerebral peduncles. The nature of the lesion is usually vascular (basilar artery thrombosis or insufficiency), but it may occasionally be traumatic or neoplastic.

Because the descending motor fibres (corticobulbar and corticospinal) are severed, the syndrome is sometimes called the 'de-efferented state'. The name 'locked-in syndrome' refers to the impossibility of action potentials leaving the brain and reaching the periphery. A third name for the condition is 'ventral pontine state' on account of the localisation of the lesion most frequently to this area. Kahn, Crosley and Schneider (1969, p. 211) used the term 'Monte Cristo syndrome' because the nineteenth-century French writer Alexandre Dumas in his novel *Count of Monte Cristo* depicted a character who was totally paralysed except for his ability to raise and lower his eyelids, and who resorted to these residual movements to communicate.

Therapy

There are no indications that locked-in syndrome patients can benefit from speech therapy. Accordingly, efforts generally aim at discovering a body part which the patient can still move freely and at designing a communication system which can efficiently implement this body part.

If the patient is able to perform some articulatory movements, technical aids are sometimes used to improve the intelligibility of speech. As an example, the case reported by Simpson, Till and Goff (1988) may be quoted. Some 21 months after onset their patient started to demonstrate spontaneous improvement in labial and lingual movements. He could again produce single monosyllables, albeit weakly and inconsistently. Some gain in intelligibility could be achieved by providing the patient with an abdominal binder, which increased the loudness of his speech output somewhat. A palatal lift was fitted to reduce air leakage through the nose, and a speech amplifier was used to further enhance speech volume.

Akinetic mutism

Patients with akinetic mutism do not move, or move very little, although they are not paralysed or have motor deficits which cannot completely account for the absence of movements.

Generally, the patients remain immobile even when exhorted to move. They do not react to noxious stimuli or else show only weak and rather ineffective reactions. However, tactile stimulation of their hand palm may elicit a grasp reflex, and peribuccal stimulation may bring about a snout reflex. Vegetative movements such as blinking, yawning and coughing may be present.

A number of patients will swallow food that is put in their mouth. However, the food may remain a long time in the oral cavity before deglutition actually takes place. There is incontinence for urine and faeces and there may be hypersomnia and a tendency to catatonia (maintenance of the positions in which the limbs or head are placed by the examiner). There often is some degree of hypo- or hypertonia, and the plantar reflex is usually extensor bilaterally. The face looks expressionless, but the eyes are open and appear lively. French neurologists therefore say that the patient evidences 'une présence oculaire', i.e. he seems to be present only through his eyes. Cairns *et al.* (1941) appropriately noted that the patient's steady gaze 'seems to give promise of speech', a promise, however, that is hardly ever fulfilled. Only very occasionally, under strong verbal stimulation, do some patients give a short answer in a weak voice or in a whisper.

Jürgens and von Cramon (1982) gave the following description of one of their patients with this severe condition:

> For somewhat more than 6 weeks, the patient remained in a state of akinetic mutism. He lay in bed nearly immobile, his eyes open most of the time, his gaze following whatever was going on in his field of vision. If stimulated strongly enough, he minimally moved his head or arms. On rare occasions, he responded to painful stimuli with a groan, but never made a semantically recognizable verbal utterance.

In some cases, however, the akinesia is not total. The patient does follow simple verbal orders but in a slow and sluggish manner. Indeed, reaction time may be as long as 2 minutes.

The patient may also spontaneously perform some simple actions which are directly related to basic needs. But here too performance is delayed. At times, as in a case reported by Klee (1961), spontaneous activity takes place only when the patient is left alone. Limited as it is, this non-verbal activity contrasts with the absence of speech.

Some patients exhibit total akinesia but for one specific motor activity. For instance, a patient of Buge *et al.* (1975), remained totally immobile except when attempts were made to feed him. Then he would actively clench his teeth. Because he could not be made to open his mouth, a nasogastric tube was placed. However, the patient tried to remove it whenever he was fed through it.

Another type of spontaneous activity was observed by Grotjahn (1936) in a boy with akinetic mutism. Although otherwise totally immobile and mute, this patient would from time to time sing a song of his own accord.

When patients recover from akinetic mutism, they may or may not remember the episode. A patient of Grotjahn (1936) who had a memory of her illness indicated that at the time she had felt indifferent and unconcerned. She had no pain and was not unhappy. She sometimes would have liked to speak or to follow the instructions she was given, but could not find the energy to do so. Acting deliberately was just beyond her. She had complete avolition. A patient described by Klee (1961) recalled that when she was mute and was stimulated verbally, 'the words were there, but they did not come'.

The patient of Cairns *et al.* (1941), on the contrary, had no memory of her episode of akinetic mutism, although while ill she had from time to time been able to whisper a monosyllabic answer or to perform a voluntary movement on order.

When patients with complete akinetic mutism start to improve, voluntary movements of the extremities usually begin to re-emerge before speech activity.

The recovery of the ability to move a limb intentionally may sometimes be used to communicate with the patient and assess some aspects of his mentation. For instance, a patient of Lhermitte *et al.* (1963) who had regained the ability to flex her arms could be instructed to use this movement to answer questions in the affirmative. Using this simple code, it was possible to ascertain that the patient understood simple spoken language and could still perform simple calculations mentally. She could also identify short written words.

When speech starts to return, articulation may be regained before phonation. For instance, the patient of Jürgens and von Cramon (1982) at first produced whispered speech. Voice returned only later.

When speech has been recovered, delivery may be normal or, on the contrary, laboured, as in the case reported by Klee (1961).

The lesion responsible for akinetic mutism may lie at various levels between the pons and the frontal lobes. Often it is found in the mesencephalic tegmentum or the periaqueductal grey matter, or in both gyri cinguli (Figure 5).

Differential diagnosis

Akinetic mutism is not always easy to diagnose. Strictly speaking only patients who do not speak and do not move (or only weakly after much stimulation), but are aware of their environment and have preserved at least elementary speech comprehension, can be said to have akinetic mutism. However, the degree of consciousness and of verbal comprehension is often very difficult to assess in patients who do not react to stimulation. That is the reason why a number of clinicians ignore awareness of the environment and speech comprehension in their diagnosis of the disease. They classify patients as having akinetic mutism if they remain mute even when stimulated and do not move either

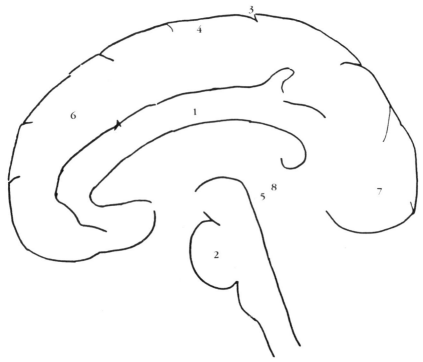

Figure 5. Sketch of a bisected brain (mesial aspect): (1) cingulate gyrus; (2) pons; (3) central sulcus; (4) supplementary motor area; (5) mesencephalic tegmentum; (6) frontal lobe; (7) occipital lobe; (8) cerebral aqueduct or aqueduct of Sylvius.

spontaneously or in reaction to external stimuli (with the possible exception of the eyes which may seem to follow movements in the room).

The problem with this diagnostic approach is that it may blur the distinction between akinetic mutism, apallism and total aphasia.

The patient with apallism (also called 'coma vigil') looks awake but does not demonstrate awareness of his environment, except for the fact that he generally reacts to painful stimuli (possibly with decerebration movements). He does not speak and does not follow verbal instructions but he may move or shout or moan spontaneously. His behaviour suggests that all his cognitive skills including language have come to a complete standstill, and that his cortex is no longer functioning. Hence the name of the condition, 'apallism', which means 'without mantle', i.e. without grey matter or cortex.

As for the patient with total (or global) aphasia, he has by definition lost the ability to use language both expressively and receptively. He is not akinetic (although he is often paralysed on one side of the body) and he is not unaware of his environment. Indeed, he usually responds adequately to non-verbal stimulation.

Although they are distinct entities, akinetic mutism, apallism and total aphasia are not always easy to keep apart in clinical practice. At times only exclusion criteria can be applied. For instance, if the patient moves or makes noises spontaneously, or if he promptly reacts to painful stimulation, he cannot be said to have akinetic mutism. If he gives an adequate verbal or gestural response to verbal stimulation (possibly after the stimulation has been repeated several times), apallism and global aphasia can be excluded. If he reacts appropriately and quickly to non-verbal innoxious stimuli, he can hardly be considered to have akinetic mutism or apallism.

Some clinicians do not clearly distinguish between akinetic mutism and the locked-in syndrome, and yet a distinction can usually be made on the basis of the state of the extremities. Patients with the locked-in syndrome have tetraplegia, whereas patients with akinetic mutism do not show signs of paralysis in their extremities or else are paralysed on only one side of the body. Moreover, catatonia may accompany akinetic mutism, whereas it virtually never co-occurs with the locked-in syndrome.

Pathophysiology

In patients with the locked-in syndrome, the corticobulbar and corticospinal fibres are massively interrupted in the ventral part of the pons or in the peduncles, and this interruption accounts for the observed symptomatology. The causal mechanism of akinetic mutism, on the contrary, is still poorly understood.

Obviously, the absence of voluntary movements in akinetic mutism is not due to paralysis as is the case with the locked-in syndrome. The musculature of patients with akinetic mutism may be hypo- or hypertonic but it is not paralysed, at least not to such an extent as needed to account for the absence of movement. What then can be the cause of akinesia in these patients? Why do they appear to lack the necessary drive to act? Where does the inhibition of voluntary movements come from?

Nielsen (1951) proposed that akinetic mutism was due to lack of affect. If a patient is completely indifferent to his environment, he has no reason to move.

There are at least two problems with this view. First, it is uncertain whether patients with akinetic mutism are totally deprived of emotion. Secondly, if it is assumed that they are, then a new, unsolved question has to be faced: Where does their complete indifference come from?

Messert, Henke and Langheim (1966) suggested that akinetic mutism represented a 'state of total apraxia involving all functions including facial expression, voice production, movements of the extremities, gait disturbances, and voluntary control of the sphincters'.

Several objections can be raised to this view. First, apraxia is by definition a disorder of deliberate movements, specifically of learned purposive movements. It does not affect reflex movements, such as retraction when painful stimulation is applied. But patients with akinetic mutism do not react, or only feebly, to noxious stimuli. These patients may also blink infrequently and may show no menace reflex, whereas in apraxic patients automatic movements and reflexes are unimpaired.

Secondly, apraxia does not as a rule clear very quickly, whereas akinetic mutism may do so occasionally. For instance, immediately after her third ventricle cyst was tapped, the patient of Cairns *et al.* (1941) 'roused and made a noise, the first loud sound she had made since admission to hospital... Within ten minutes, she gave her name, age, and address correctly without any trace of dysarthria, and then asked where she was. She co-operated perfectly in an examination'. Such sudden recovery is generally not observed in patients with apraxia.

These patients also do not show episodes of unimpaired performance, whereas this may sometimes be observed in akinetic mutism. For instance, a young woman with akinetic mutism mentioned by Klee (1961) could become 'for some minutes nearly normal in speech, movement and expression'.

For these various reasons it is difficult to construe the absence of movement in akinetic mutism as total apraxia.

Maybe the akinesia in this syndrome should be viewed as resulting from an inhibition of motor centres. Where this inhibition comes from is not clear, however. Klee (1961) suggested that it might result from a disturbance of the coordinating centrencephalic system postulated by Penfield and Jasper (1954). But what the role of this hypothetical centre exactly is and how it can be impaired are still highly conjectural.

Reports of improvement of akinetic mutism under the influence of pharmacological treatment (Daly and Love, 1958; Ross and Stewart, 1981) raise the question of whether in some cases the condition might not be the result of a disturbance of one or more of the different neurotransmitter systems. However, in cases where akinetic mutism was suddenly alleviated (as in the girl described by Cairns *et al*, 1941), a neurotransmitter disorder can hardly be assumed. Probably in such instances a mechanical compression of the motor system has to be presumed. This compression may at times be due to obstructive hydrocephalus, as suggested by Messert, Henke and Langheim (1966).

In summary, the pathophysiology of akinetic mutism remains obscure. Probably the condition can be precipitated by various factors. This hypothesis is consistent with the observation that the causal lesion may lie at different levels of the central nervous system.

Hyperkinetic mutism

Under the title 'hyperkinetic mutism' Inbody and Jankovic (1986) described a woman who, in addition to being mute, had continuous coarse, bilateral, ballistic movements of arms and legs with choreic movements of hand and fingers and oromandibular and lingual dyskinesia. Except for her bilateral ballism, which ceased during sleep, she resembled patients with akinetic mutism: she seemed alert and her eyes moved in a conjugate, roving manner as if she were visually following objects and people in the room. She withdrew and grimaced in response to painful stimuli. Otherwise, she did not react to stimulation and did not speak. Neuroradiology documented bilateral basal ganglia calcification and bilateral parieto-occipital infarcts.

In a woman with mutism and hypokinesia and whose comprehension of simple speech was preserved, Serdaru, Lechevalier and Gray (1982) observed severe myoclonias of the right arm and to some extent also of the right leg. These involuntary muscle contractions occurred when the patient was touched or stimulated.

Traut (1935) reported the case of a young woman who, after a prolonged state of stupor accompanied by high fever and rigidity, showed akinetic mutism concomitant with involuntary clonic muscular contractions. Traut noted that 'these convulsive movements were often marked enough to throw her out of bed'.

Akinetic mutism may therefore be accompanied by unintentional movements which stand in contrast to the overall immobility or the absence of voluntary movements.

Therapy

A number of clinicians including Gouazé, Lebatard and Rolland (1977) recommend giving patients with akinetic mutism sustained verbal stimulation with a view to accelerating recovery of verbal (re)activity. They suggest showing the patient familiar photographs or familiar objects (such as tools he uses professionally) and adding copious verbal comment to each item shown. They also advise singing songs known to the patient in the hope that he might join in at some point. Finally, they indicate that wrong affective statements made on purpose may be useful in eliciting an emotional reaction possibly accompanied or followed by words.

If the patient is not totally akinetic he should be encouraged to move more frequently, to act purposely, to make noises and later to produce speech sounds, and also to write, first with anagram letters and later using pen and paper.

Mutism following surgery in the fossa posterior

In 1980 Pierre-Kahn et al. briefly mentioned 10 children who had had fossa posterior surgery, as a consequence of which they had transient mutism without akinesia. Mutism tended not to present immediately after surgery; it generally appeared a few days later, and it disappeared spontaneously after some time.

These observations were confirmed by Rekate *et al.* (1985) who reported six children who had been mute following surgery involving the cerebellar vermis, the cerebellar hemispheres and the deep nuclei of the cerebellum. In all six cases muteness resolved over a period of 1–3 months and was followed by cerebellar dysarthria.

In one case, which is described in some detail, the patient initially did not swallow although the gag reflex was present. A little later, spontaneous movements of lip, tongue and velum returned. Six weeks after surgery she started to produce voice during laughing and crying. By 3 months expressive speech had been recovered but there was dysarthria.

Another case of mutism in a child following fossa posterior surgery was reported by Volcan, Cole and Johnston (1986). Mutism lasted for 2 weeks. It was not accompanied by dysphagia, and spontaneous whining was present.

It is not clear whether this type of mutism should be interpreted as a specific kind of 'muteness of cerebellar origin' (Rekate *et al.*, 1985) or whether its cause should be looked for in the midbrain (Pierre-Kahn *et al.*, 1980). In point of fact, mutism has repeatedly been observed following mesencephalic lesions and it was often accompanied by akinesia (e.g. Grotjahn, 1936; Cairns *et al.*, 1941; Cairns, 1952; Brage, Morea and Copello, 1961; Lhermitte *et al.*, 1963; Messert, Henke and Langheim, 1966). But in a few cases, there was no concomitant akinesia (e.g. Cairns, 1952; Daly and Lowe, 1958). The kind of mutism reported by Pierre-Kahn *et al.* (1980), Rekate *et al.* (1985) and Volcan *et al.* (1986) may therefore belong to this latter group.

Parkinsonism

In a number of patients with Parkinson's disease, hypokinesia and hypertonia are so pronounced that speech movements become impossible. For the same reason, the patients may be unable to write, or else produce micrographia. However, comprehension of ordinary verbal messages is preserved.

Under the influence of a strong affect, these mute patients may suddenly become able to utter a few sentences. They may also occasionally be heard to speak during sleep.

Not only emotion or sleep but also paroxysmal brain activity may at times relieve mutism. For instance, Van Bogaert (1934) observed a man who had postencephalitic parkinsonism with complete mutism. Now and then, he also had speech comprehension difficulties and, moreover, he had epileptic fits with oculogyric movements. During these fits he was able to express himself orally. However, some of his utterances, especially at the beginning of the paroxysmal spells, were palilalic.

Speech therapy seems to have little influence on the speechlessness of hypokinetic and hypertonic parkinsonian patients. For instance, Wunderli (1962) described a 25-year-old female with postencephalitic parkinsonism. She could no longer speak and could only slowly move her extremities. Although small her writing was legible. She communicated in writing and by means of drawings. She was given speech therapy but to no avail. Electrocoagulation of the right pallidum internum also failed to bring about any improvement.

Paradoxical mutism

A number of patients with parkinsonian symptoms have intermittent mutism. Sometimes they can speak freely; at other times, despite their desire to communicate orally, they are unable to activate their speech organs. This intermittent speechlessness, which Souques (cited in Babinski, Jarkowski and Plichet, 1921) proposed to call 'paradoxical mutism', occurs primarily when the patient is about to speak deliberately. Ejaculations of words under the influence of strong affects are generally unimpaired. Indeed, a sudden emotion may put an end to a spell of mutism.

Speech activities such as repetition, reading aloud and recitation, which are less creative than spontaneous speech, may be possible whilst self-expression is inhibited. Actually, engaging the patient in repetition may enable him to speak spontaneously for some time. Paradoxical mutism therefore has features that are reminiscent of Hughlings Jackson's distinction between propositional and automatic speech.

When the patient goes through a spell of mutism he may, as in the case reported by Babinski, Jarkowski and Plichet (1921), be unable to open his mouth on request or to eat. He may even be drooling because he fails to swallow his saliva. Indeed, in some cases, paradoxical mutism is accompanied by pronounced overall hypokinesia.

When the episode is over, the patient generally explains that he was all the time trying to speak but could not make his articulators move. Generally the patient's efforts to speak are not perceptible to an observer.

Commissurotomy

Mutism may also be observed after commissurotomy. For instance, Bogen and Vogel (1975) found temporary mutism immediately following surgery in a number of patients who had undergone transection of the corpus callosum for intractable epilepsy. The authors reported that 'there was in almost every case a postoperative period of mutism, of varying duration, during which speech was absent or extremely sparse, although comprehension and writing were retained'. Before speech completely normalised some patients went through a stage of hoarseness or whispering.

In one case, mutism was still present several years after surgery. It was very seldomly interrupted by an occasional utterance spoken in a husky voice. The patient also had some degree of oral apraxia.

Mutism of 16 months' duration was noted by Sussman *et al.* (1983) in a young man who had undergone callosotomy at the age of 18. During this 16 month period, only eight brief one-sentence outbursts of speech were heard. Mutism was concomitant with severe oral apraxia. The patient comprehended oral and written language and expressed himself in writing or by means of gestures.

Sixteen months after operation he started to whisper. Then voice was recovered, but it was breathy. Articulation was laborious, and oral apraxia had not totally disappeared.

The pathophysiology of postcommissurotomy mutism is still poorly understood. It is not clear whether the speechlessness is a direct consequence of the trans-section of the callosal fibres or, on the contrary, a result of diaschisis.

Speech arrests

Epilepsy

During epileptic fits without loss of consciousness (so-called 'partial seizures') patients may be deprived of the ability to express themselves orally. For instance, Barris and Schuman (1953) described a patient who had periods of jerking in his right lower limb. During these jacksonian fits he was 'neither able to reply to questions nor capable of spontaneous speech'.

Such paroxysmal suspensions of spoken language with preservation of verbal comprehension are usually called 'speech arrests'. Strenuous efforts on the part of the patient to speak during them generally result only in a few indistinct sounds.

At the beginning of the seizure, the patient may involuntarily produce a protracted sound or repeat a sound several times before losing his faculty of speech. However, at the end of the episode causing speech arrest, he may be able to repeat somebody's words whilst still unable to speak spontaneously.

As an instance of ictal speech arrest, the case reported by Vernea (1974) may be quoted. The patient had chronic epilepsy. Paroxysmal activity could be partially controlled by medication. One day the patient had a series of partial seizures following each other in quick succession. This 'status epilepticus' lasted for about 2 hours. During this period of time the patient understood what he was told. He could perform even complex orders, whether they were given orally or in writing. On request he could write words and sentences. He could also open and close his mouth and eyes, move his tongue and show his teeth. He could deliberately modify his respiratory pattern. However, he was totally unable to speak or, indeed, to produce any vocal sound.

Not infrequently, paroxysmal speech arrests are caused by a tumour invading or compressing the upper mesial aspect of the frontal lobe. For instance, in a case reported by Guidetti (1957), a meningioma of the falx cerebri which pressed on the posterior part of the mesial surface of the left frontal lobe induced epileptic fits during which the patient was unable to speak and write but could follow simple verbal instructions. At the beginning of each episode, before becoming mute, the patient involuntarily let out a sustained yell.

Botez and Wertheim (1959) have reported the case of a right-handed male who had partial epileptic fits caused by a tumour in the posterior third of the first two frontal convolutions on the right. During these seizures, he remained conscious and could understand what he was told. But he could not speak. At times, instead of being mute, he would involuntarily produce a palilalic series of speech sounds.

In the case reported by Lebrun (1976) and mentioned on p. 84, the paroxysmal speech arrests were caused by a meningioma compressing the left operculum Rolandi.

Occasionally verbal comprehension appears somewhat impaired during the epileptic fits, as in a case observed by Gilmore and Heilman (1981). The speech arrest is then a component of paroxysmal motor aphasia.

Peled *et al.* (1984) have reported a case in which not only speech but also writing was precluded during seizures. It is not clear whether the disturbance of writing was aphasic in nature or due to a paroxysmal inhibition of graphomotricity.

It appears therefore that paroxysmal mutism may be pure or, on the contrary, may be accompanied by some degree of aphasia.

Migraine

In 1979 Jenkyn and Reeves described a female patient who showed speech arrests during migrainous episodes. Suspension of speech was concomitant with monoplegia of the right leg. The transitory speechlessness was pure in the sense that the patient could express herself in writing, and her comprehension of spoken and written language was unimpaired, at least at the clinical level. No formal aphasia examination was performed, which perhaps would have disclosed slight linguistic deficits during the migrainous spells.

Electrical stimulation

Speech arrests may also occur following electrical stimulation of some cerebral structure. The patient is requested to count orally, to recite something he knows by heart or to name the pictures he is shown. At some point in the verbal performance, an electric current is applied across a group of cerebral neurones. This electrical stimulation may interrupt the verbal action, causing an involuntary arrest of speech. Usually, the patient is able to resume the verbal task as soon as the stimulation ceases.

Generally, verbal comprehension is maintained during the provoked speech arrest. When electrical stimulation ceased, a patient who had been prevented from answering the surgeon's questions, said: 'I could hear what you were saying, doctor. I knew what I wanted to say but just couldn't' (Penfield and Welch, 1951).

Speech arrests of this type have been observed following electrical stimulation of the cortex (Penfield and Roberts, 1959) and of subcortical structures, particularly the thalamus (Ojemann, 1976).

Penfield and Rasmussen (1949) found that speech interference resulted with equal frequency from electrical stimulation of the right and of the left sensorimotor cortex, and Ojemann (1976) observed no difference between the right and left side during electrical stimulation of the thalamus resulting in speech arrest. These experimental findings should probably be related to the clinical observation that mutism can result from a lesion in the right as well as from a lesion in the left hemisphere (see p. 77).

Penfield and Rasmussen (1949) and Penfield and Welch (1951) found that speech interference could also result from electrical stimulation of the supplementary motor cortex in the upper and mesial part of either frontal lobe. This finding is reminiscent not only of the case reported by Guidetti (1957) where a tumour near the supplementary motor cortex caused paroxysmal speech arrests (see p. 99), but also of the case reported by Petit-Dutaillis *et al.* (1954) where a bleeding aneurysm located in that area rendered the patient mute (see p. 78).

Intoxication

Marcotte (1972) described a temporary inability to speak in four patients who had been smoking marijuana. However, it is not clear from his description whether comprehension of speech was preserved during the episode of mutism. One of the patients did report that during his spell of speechlessness he had been 'confused and unable to follow their [his companions] statements accurately'. This remark suggests that comprehension of speech was impaired but it is uncertain to what degree. In none of the four cases was writing tested during the episode of speechlessness. Accordingly, it is still not settled whether inhalation of marijuana can cause transient pure mutism or temporary aphasia with total loss of the ability to speak, i.e. transient aphasic mutism.

Cataplexy

Cataplexy is an affection that manifests itself in fits, which are usually precipitated by some emotion, such as mirth or excitement.

Although he is not paralysed, the patient is unable to voluntarily contract a number of muscles during the cataleptic fit. If the affected muscles are those of speech, he cannot talk. If the musculature of the upper extremities is also involved, he is equally unable to write. Although he cannot express himself, the patient remains fully conscious and his comprehension of speech is intact.

Some authors use the words 'catalepsy' or 'narcolepsy' to refer to this condition.

Narcolepsy

The term 'narcolepsy' is in fact more appropriately applied to a disorder characterised by bouts of sleepiness.

A patient of Botez (1964), who suffered from narcolepsy, could often avoid falling asleep by starting to walk when he felt that a seizure was coming on. But for 5–10 minutes he was unable to speak.

Various factors may therefore temporarily inhibit the cerebral speech production mechanisms whilst leaving the other verbal skills of the patient unabated or at least largely preserved. The cause of such speech arrests may be diffuse or lateralised to one hemisphere.

Speech apraxia

Mutism without paralytic impairment of the speech musculature may at times be observed in the initial stage of apraxia of speech. Immediately following onset the apraxia of the speech organs may be so severe that the patient is unable to say a single word. Indeed, sometimes not even a single speech sound can be uttered. For instance, Lebrun (1976) described a patient who was a foreman in a factory. One night, he was assailed by hooligans. He received several blows on the head, one of them causing a left temporoparietal fracture. The patient was taken to hospital. He was conscious but could not speak. He resorted to writing to express himself. What he wrote was quite intelligible despite some substitutions and omissions of letters. He was trepanned and his cerebral wound cleansed.

Four days after surgery the patient was fully conscious but totally speechless. All his attempts at speaking resulted in unintelligible grunts. There was no paralysis of the speech musculature, no oral apraxia and no dysphagia. Comprehension of spoken and written language was normal. The patient expressed himself by means of grimaces and gestures and also by means of written language. Apart from a few spelling errors, his written output was correct and appropriate. A few days later, speech started to return. The patient at first uttered isolated speech sounds, then isolated short words, and finally polysyllabic words and short sentences. His articulation was grossly deviant.

Internal language competence

A few days after surgery, when he was still totally unable to utter speech sounds, let alone to speak, the patient of Lebrun (1976) was given metalinguistic tasks requiring him to manipulate the phonology of French, his mother-tongue. For instance, he was shown a series of everyday objects and asked to point to the objects in the series whose names began with the same sound. The patient made no error on such tests.

A similar observation was made by Nebes (1975). Following a stroke in the left hemisphere his patient became speechless whilst retaining the ability to express herself in writing and to understand both spoken and written language. Despite her total inability to speak, this woman performed normally on tasks requiring her to find, in a series of objects, the object whose name rhymed with the name of an object presented separately, or to find in a list of written words the word that rhymed with a written word presented separately. She succeeded in the latter task even when the two words had different spellings (e.g. 'new' and 'through') and there were foils such as 'mouth' and 'trough' in the list.

Motor theory of speech perception

The findings of Lebrun (1976) and Nebes (1975) mentioned above may be compared with the observations made by Vallar and Cappa (1987) in a case of locked-in syndrome (see p. 88). Although a pontine lesion had rendered him totally mute, the patient of Vallar and Cappa could in a series of four pictures indicate the one whose name rhymed with the name of a given picture shown separately or with a given word presented orally. He could also discriminate between similar nonsense syllables such as /ba/, /da/, /ga/, /pa/, /ta/ and /ka/.

These various test results show that the loss of articulate speech following brain damage does not necessarily prevent the patient from evoking and processing phonological components of language. This holds true even in cases where the lesion is primarily cortical and disturbs the programming of articulatory movements, as in speech apraxia.

As was pointed out by Lebrun (1970), preservation of verbal comprehension and of internal speech in patients with complete loss of articulatory abilities casts strong doubts on the validity of the motor theory of speech perception. According to this theory, speech is understood by reference to articulation, i.e. the listener has to reproduce the words he hears before he can understand them. The kinaesthetic feedback he obtains from his articulatory movements enables him to decode the perceived message (Lieberman, 1957; Denes, 1967).

The clinical cases discussed above show that, contrary to this theory, verbal comprehension does not depend on the ability to articulate. Indeed, it does not seem to require any kinaesthetic feedback at all. Furthermore, the ability to make judgements based on the manipulation of phonology may remain unabated even if articulatory skills are lost.

Differential diagnosis

In speech apraxia complete mutism is typically transient. After a few days, possibly a few weeks, the patient starts to utter sounds again and, after a little while, words. If mutism lasts longer, the diagnosis of speech apraxia may be questioned. The patient is likely to have a different affection, possibly motor aphasia.

Some speech pathologists disagree with the claim made here that persistent mutism is not characteristic of speech apraxia. They oppose this view because they regard speech apraxia as a frequent accompaniment of (motor) aphasia rather than as an independent syndrome.

If speech apraxia is separated from motor aphasia, as sound nosology seems to require (Lebrun, 1982, 1989), then the mutism which may sometimes be present at the onset of speech apraxia typically proves to be of short duration. This is in line with the observation that apraxia generally prevents a patient not from making gestures but from performing the appropriate movements and/or from performing them in the proper order.

In motor aphasia, on the contrary, the absence of oral–verbal output can be a persistent deficit. However, even if he is totally mute, the patient with motor aphasia may be able to sing, i.e. he may be capable of producing words when they are embedded in a familiar melody, as a case reported by Keith and Aronson (1975) shows.

According to Benton and Joynt (1960) the dissociation between speaking and singing in motor aphasia was recorded as early as the eighteenth century by a Swede, Olof Dalin, who described 'a mute who could sing'. In speech apraxia, on the contrary, words cannot be better produced in singing than in speech, as was already pointed out by Dejerine in 1901 (Dejerine, however, did not use the label 'speech apraxia' but spoke of 'pure motor aphasia', which he, quite appropriately, contrasted with 'cortical motor aphasia', i.e. 'Broca's aphasia').

When speech returns in patients with speech apraxia, it is severely distorted and usually remains so for months if not for years. Indeed, articulation may never fully normalise. If the patient proves to have correct articulation and fluent delivery when mutism clears up, the diagnosis of speech apraxia should be questioned. Most probably the patient suffered from some inhibition of his speech production mechanism which was not apraxic in nature.

Initially, when the patient is completely mute, differential diagnosis may be difficult. Due to the fact that immediately following onset apraxia of speech may be accompanied by unilateral motor weakness and by some degree of agraphia (probably as a result of diaschisis), it may be impossible to decide whether the patient actually has complete apraxia of speech, mutism accompanied by a pyramidal hemisyndrome (see p. 75) or aphasic mutism (see p. 83).

Conclusions

There seems to be no other human behaviour which can be suspended by a lesion in so many different parts of the central nervous system as speaking. From the cortex down to the neuromuscular junction, a variety of injuries can render a patient mute. However, it is not always clear how the damage suffered by the nervous system interferes with speech production.

At times the pyramidal tract is injured directly and bilaterally. It is then easy to understand the resulting paralysis and the loss of speech movements. Mutism in pseudobulbar palsy, the opercular syndrome, the locked-in syndrome or diseases of the motor neurones is not difficult to explain.

On the contrary, mutism following injury to only one side of the pyramidal tract is surprising. Why does the voluntary innervation of the speech organs, which have bilateral nerve supply, sometimes break down completely following unilateral hemispherical damage? How is mutism concomitant with a pyramidal hemisyndrome to be accounted for? Are activation and control of the vocal tract so fully integrated that damage to one side of its dual driving system is sufficient to put the whole system out of order? It looks as if this is actually the case.

Absence of speech in patients with severe hypokinesia and hypertonia of extrapyramidal origin is comprehensible. More puzzling is so-called paradoxical mutism. What is the cause of this intermittent mutism which in some cases appears to depend on the propositionality of speech?

The pathophysiology of akinetic mutism or mutism following commissurotomy (especially when the duration of the speechlessness exceeds normal diaschisis) is no less perplexing.

Probably, meaningful speech production requires the precise integration of so many different cerebral functions, and the harmonious participation of so many neuronal subsets, that disturbance of one or a few of these functions, or disruption of one or a few of these subsets, is sufficient at times to jam the whole mechanism and render the patient mute. Some of these functions and their anatomical substrates are well known, others are still largely mysterious.

Epilogue

Each form of mutism has a fascination of its own. Whether functional or organic, selective or total, intermittent or permanent, the absence or suspension of expressive speech is intriguing and disconcerting.

Functional mutism astonishes both with its motives and with its constancy. It is amazing that someone should be unable to bring himself to interact with others through the spoken word. Oral–verbal intercourse seems so natural, so congenial to man, that the prolonged inhibition of expressive speech appears weird and baffling. Each of us can remember so many occasions when he should have held his peace but was unable to do so and gave himself away, that we cannot help marvelling at the sustained silence of the functionally mute individual, a silence which resists all punishments, withstands seduction and often outwits even the most able of therapists.

At the same time, functional mutism irritates us. In its presence we feel cheated and denied. We consider ourselves entitled to a verbal response, and we resent getting none. Praiseworthy as it may be, silence should not be permanent. Humans are expected to be verbal, even though they should not be verbose. Mutes, we feel, are like zombies. They are estranged from themselves and from the others. Therefore, their condition should be changed and speech reinstated, whenever possible. Permanent speechlessness is an evil which society has a right to combat.

Organic mutism too should be fought. The patient afflicted with it is a prisoner within himself, and he needs to be freed.

Because they are deprived of expressive speech, patients with organic mutism stir up our sympathy. We have compassion for them. They are immured in silence and unable to express themselves, to fight for themselves, indeed to be themselves. Speech is so much part of our human inheritance that the loss of it endangers the integrity of self. One day, French essayist Valéry Larbaud who had been rendered almost mute by a cerebrovascular accident, met friends who enquired how he was doing.

Valéry Larbaud could only give a one-word response, but this one word conveyed all his desperation: 'Déchu', i.e. downfallen (Lebrun, 1978a).

As a disease, organic mutism is frequently perplexing. We often find it hard to understand why a patient can no longer speak. At times, the central speech mechanism gets blocked for reasons which are not at all clear. More than once, involuntary silence cannot be explained.

Mutism is like a sphinx — it is both captivating and disquieting. It stares at us defiantly, and we find it difficult to solve its silent riddle. Language pathology has not produced its Oedipus yet, and the enigma of muteness remains largely hidden.

References

ABRAHAM, S. and LLEWELLYN-JONES, D. (1984). *Eating Disorders*. Oxford: Oxford University Press.

ADAMS, H. and GLASSNER, P. (1954). Emotional involvement in some forms of mutism. *Journal of Speech and Hearing Disorders* 19: 59–69.

AJURIAGUERRA, (DE) J. (1977). *Manuel de psychiatrie de l'enfant*. Paris: Masson.

AJURIAGUERRA, J., DIAKTINE, R. and DE GOBINEAU, H. (1956). L'écriture en miroir. *Semaine des Hôpitaux de Paris* 32: 80–86.

AKHTAR, S. and BUCKMAN, J. (1977). The differential diagnosis of mutism: A review and a report of three unusual cases. *Diseases of the Nervous System* 38: 558–562.

ALAJOUANINE, T. and THUREL, R. (1933). La diplégie faciale cérébrale, forme corticale de la paralysise pseudo-bulbaire. *Revue Neurologique* 2: 411–458.

ALAJOUANINE, T., BOUDIN, G., PERTUISET, B. and PEPIN, B. (1959a). Le syndrome operculaire unilatéral avec atteinte contralatérale du territoire des V, VII, IX, X, XI, XIIe neris crâniens. *Revue Neurologique* 101: 168–171.

ALAJOUANINE, T., LHERMITTE, F., CAMBIER, J., RONDOT, P. and LEFEBVRE, J. (1959b). Perturbations dissociées de la motricité facio-bucco-pharyngée avec aphémie dans un ramollisement sylvien profond partiel. *Revue Neurologique* 101: 493–498.

ALTSHULER, L., CUMMINGS, J. and MILLS, M. (1987). Reply to David. *American Journal of Psychiatry* 144: 1113.

ARNOLD, G. (1948). *Die traumatischen und konstitutionellen Störungen der Stimme und Sprache*. Vienna: Urban und Schwarzenberg.

BABINSKI, J. (1904). Introduction à la sémiologie des affections du système nerveux. *Gazette des Hôpitaux* Oct. 11.

BABINSKI, J., JARKOWSKI, B. and PLICHET (1921). Kinésie paradoxale. Mutisme parkinsonien. *Revue Neurologique* 28: 1266–1270.

BACH, J. (1890). Hysterical aphonia. *Medical News* 57 (Sept. 13): 263–264.

BAK, E., VAN DONGEN, H. and ARTS, W. (1983). The analysis of acquired dysarthria in childhood. *Developmental Medicine and Child Neurology* 25: 81–94.

BARRIS, R. and SCHUMAN, H. (1953). Bilateral anterior cingulate gyrus lesions. *Neurology* 3: 44–52.

BARTON, R. (1965). A review of attempted physiological restoration of voice following total laryngectomy. *Proceedings of the Eighth International Congress of Otorhinolaryngology*, Tokyo, pp. 731–734.

BASSO, K. (1970). To give up on words: Silence in the Western Apache culture. In Giglioli P. (Ed.) *Language and Social Context*. Harmondsworth: Penguin.

107

BAUERMEISTER, J. and JEMAIL, J. (1975). Modification of 'elective mutism' in the classroom setting: A case study. *Behavior Therapy* **6**: 246–250.

BEDNAR, R. (1974). A behavioral approach to treating an elective mute in the school. *Journal of School Psychology* **12**: 326–337.

BENTON, A. and JOYNT, R. (1960). Early description of aphasia. *Archives of Neurology* **3**: 205–222.

BERTHIER, M., STARKSTEIN, S. and LEIGUARDA, R. (1987). Behavioral effects of damage to the right insula and surrounding regions. *Cortex* **23**: 673–678.

BITTORF, A. (1915). Zur Behandlung der nach Granatexplosionen auftretenden Neurosen. *Münchener medizinische Wochenschrift* **30**: 1029–1030.

BLOTCKY, M. and LOONEY, J. (1980). A psychotherapeutic approach to silent children. *American Journal of Psychotherapy* **24**: 487–495.

BOGEN, J. and VOGEL, P. (1975). Neurological status in the long term following complete cerebral commissurotomy. In Michel, F. and Schott, B. (Eds) *Les syndromes de disconnexion calleuse chez l'homme*, pp. 227–252, Lyon.

BOTEZ, M. (1964). The starting mechanism of speech. *Ideggyogyaszati* **1**: 13–29.

BOTEZ, M. and WERTHEIM, N. (1959). Expressive aphasia and amusia. *Brain* **82**: 186–202.

BOUDIN, G., PEPIN, B. and WIART, J. (1960). Le syndrome operculaire unilatéral d'origine vasculaire. *Revue Neurologique* **103**: 65.

BRADLEY, S. and SLOMAN, L. (1975). Elective mutism in immigrant families. *Journal of the American Academy of Child Psychiatry* **14**: 510–514.

BRAGE, D., MOREA, R. and COPELLO, A. (1961). Syndrome nécrotique tegmento-thalamique avec mutisme akinétique. *Revue Neurologique* **104**: 126–137.

BRISON, D. (1966). Case studies in school psychology. A non-talking child in kindergarten: An application of behavior therapy. *Journal of School Psychology* **4**: 65–69.

BROCA, P. (1861). Remarques sur le siège de la faculté de langage suivies d'une observation d'aphémie. *Bulletin de la Société d'Anatomie* **6**: 330–357.

BROWN, W. (1918). The treatment of cases of shell shock in an advanced neurological centre. *Lancet* August 17: 197–200.

BUGE, A., ESCOUROLLE, R., RANCUREL, G. and POISSON, M. (1975). Mutisme akinétique et ramollissement bi-cingulaire. *Revue Neurologique* **131**: 121–137.

CAIRNS, H. (1952). Disturbances of consciousness with lesions of the brain-stem and diencephalon. *Brain* **75**: 109–146.

CAIRNS, H., OLDFIELD, R., PENNYBACKER, J. and WHITTERIDGE, D. (1941). Akinetic mutism with an epidermoid cyst of the third ventricle. *Brain* **64**: 273–290.

CAPPA, S., PRIROVANO, C. and VIGNOLO, L. (1985). Chronic 'locked-in' syndrome: Psychological study of a case. *European Neurology* **24**: 107–111.

CAPPA, S., GUIDOTTI, M., PAPAGNO, C. and VIGNOLO, L. (1987). Speechlessness with occasional vocalizations after bilateral opercular lesions: A case study. *Aphasiology* **1**: 35–40.

CHATEAU, R., FAU, R., GROSLAMBERT, R., PERRET, J., BOUCHARLAT, J. and CHATELAIN, R. (1966). A propos de trois observations de diplégie linguo-facio-masticatrice d'origine corticale: la forme de l'adulte et celle de l'enfant. *Revue Neurologique* **114**: 390–395.

CHETHIK, M. (1977). Amy: The intensive treatment of an elective mute. In MacDermott, J. and Harrison, S. (Eds) *Psychiatric Treatment of the Child*, pp. 117–136. New York: Aronson.

CHIA, L. and KINSBOURNE, M. (1987). Mirror-writing and reversed repetition of digits in a right-handed patient with left basal ganglia hematoma. *Journal of Neurology, Neurosurgery and Psychiatry* **50**: 786–788.

COLLIGAN, R., COLLIGAN, R. and DILLIARD, M. (1977). Contingency management in the classroom treatment of long-term elective mutism: A case report. *Journal of School Psychology* **15**: 9–17.

CRITCHLEY, M. (1970). *Aphasiology and Other Aspects of Language.* London: Arnold.

CUMMINGS, J., BENSON, F., HOULIHAN, J. and GOSENFELD, L. (1983). Mutism: Loss of neocortical and limbic vocalization. *Journal of Nervous and Mental Disease* **171**: 255–259.

DALY, D. and LOVE, G. (1958). Akinetic mutism. *Neurology* **8**: 238–242.

DAMASIO, A., DAMASIO, H., RIZZO, M., VARNEY, N. and GERSH, F. (1982). Aphasia with nonhemorrhagic lesions in the basal ganglia and internal capsule. *Archives of Neurology* **39**: 15–20.

D'AMBROSIO, R. (1970). *No Language but a Cry.* New York: Dell

DAVID, A. and BONE, I. (1984). Mutism following left hemisphere infarction. *Journal of Neurology, Neurosurgery and Psychiatry* **47**: 1342–1344.

DE BRUINE GROENEVELDT (1924). De spraek na larynxexstirpatie. *Nederlands Tijdschrift voor Geneeskunde* **68**, 2A: 1448–1449.

DEJERINE, J. (1901). Sémiologie du système nerveux nerveux. In Bouchard (Ed.) *Traité de pathologie générale*, vol. 5, 391–471. Paris: Masson.

DE MOL, J. and DELEVAL, J. (1979). Le mutisme post-traumatique. *Acta Neurologica Belgica* **79**: 369–383.

DE MORSIER, G. (1949). Les troubles de la déglutition et des mouvements de la langue dans l'anarthrie (aphasie motrice). *Practica Oto-Rhino-Laryngologica* **11**: 125–133.

DE MORSIER, G. (1973). Sur 23 cas d'aphasie traumatique *Psychiatria Clinica* 6: 226–239.

DENES, B. (1967). On the motor theory of speech perception. In Wathen-Dunn, W. (Ed.) *Models for the Perception of Speech and Visual Form*, pp. 309–314. Cambridge: MIT Press.

DOMS, M. (1976). A case of mutism resistant to speech therapy. In Lebrun, Y. and Hoops, R. (Eds) *Recovery in Aphasics*, pp. 54–56. Amsterdam: Swets & Zeitlinger.

DUGAS, M., VELIN, J., GUERIOT, C. and CARBONELL, L. (1972). Mutisme et faux mutisme chez l'enfant. *Concours Médical* **94** (48): 8173–8183.

EITINGER, L. (1953). Aphonia: Is aphonia always a hysterical symptom? *Acta Psychiatrica et Neurologica* **27/28**: 27–34.

ELLES, G. (1962). The mute sad-eyed child: Collateral analysis in a disturbed family. *International Journal of Psycho-Analysis* **43**: 40–49.

ELLIOTT, D. and NEEDLEMAN, R. (1976). The syndrome of hyperlexia. *Brain and Language* **3**: 339–349.

ELSON, A., PEARSON, C., JONES, D. and SCHUMACHER, E. (1965). Follow-up study of childhood elective mutism. *Archives of General Psychiatry* **13**: 182–187.

FOURCIN, A. (1975). Language development in the absence of expressive speech. In Lenneberg, F. (Ed.) *Foundations of Language Development II*, pp. 263–268. New York: Academic Press.

GARGAN, W. (1969). *Why Me?* New York: Doubleday.

GAROUX, R., LOMBERTIE, E., DUMOND, J., MALAUZAT, D. and LEGER, J. (1982). A propos d'un cas de mutisme. *Actualités Psychiatriques* **8**: 108–111.

GAUGER, G. (1980). Communication in the locked-in syndrome. *Transactions of the American Society for Artificial Internal Organs* **26**: 527–529.

GILMORE, R. and HEILMAN, K. (1981). Speech arrests in partial seizures: Evidence of an associated language disorder. *Neurology* **31**: 1016–1019.

GOLDSTEIN, M. (1940). Speech without a tongue. *Journal of Speech Disorders* **5**: 65–70

GOLL, K. (1979). Role structure and subculture in families of elective mutists. *Family Proceedings* **18**: 55–68.

GOUAZE, V., LEBATARD, M. and ROLLAND, J. (1977). Le mutisme akinétique et le mutisme post-contusionnel: rôle de l'orthophoniste. *Revue de Laryngologie* **98**: 123–128.

GROSSWASSER, Z., KORN, C., GROSSWASSER-REIDER, I. and SOLZI, P. (1988). Mutism associated with bucco-facial apraxia and bihemispheric lesions. *Brain and Language* **34**: 157–168.

GROTJAHN, M. (1936). Klinik und Bedeutung akinetischer Zustände nach Luftfüllung des dritten Ventrikels. *Monatsschrift für Psychiatrie und Neurologie* **93**: 121–139.

GUIDETTI, B. (1957). Désordres de la parole associés à des lésions de la surface interhémisphérique frontale postérieure. *Revue Neurologique* **97**: 121–131.

GUTTMANN, E. (1942). Aphasia in children. *Brain* **65**: 205–219.

GUTZMANN, H. (1959). Ueber psychogene Aphonien. *Archiv für Ohren-, Nasen- und Kehlkopfheilkunde* **175**: 437–441.

HALPERN, W., HAMMOND, J. and COHEN, R. (1971). A therapeutic approach to speech phobia: Elective mutism reexamined. *Journal of the American Academy of Child Psychiatry* **10**: 94–107.

HAYAKAWA, S. (1964). *Language in Thought and Action.* New York: Harcourt, Brace and World.

HAYDEN, T. (1980). Classification of elective mutism. *Journal of the American Academy of Child Psychiatry* **19**: 118–133.

HAYDEN, T. (1983). *Murphy's Boy.* New York: Putnam.

HEAD, H. (1926). *Aphasia and Kindred Disorders of Speech.* Cambridge: Cambridge University Press.

HILL, L. and SCULL, J. (1985). Elective mutism associated with selective inactivity. *Journal of Communication Disorders* **18**: 161–167.

HIRSCHFELD, R. (1916). Zur Behandlung im Kriege erworbener hysterischer Zustände, insbesondere von Sprachstörungen. *Zeitschrift für die gesamte Neurologie und Psychiatrie* **34**: 195–205.

INBODY, S. and JANKOVIC, J. (1986). Hyperkinetic mutism: Bilateral ballism and basal ganglia calcification. *Neurology* **36**: 825–827.

ISAACS, W., THOMAS, J. and GOLDIAMOND, I. (1960). Application of operant conditioning to reinstate verbal behavior in psychotics. *Journal of Speech and Hearing Disorders* **25**: 8–12.

ITARD, J. (1801, 1807). *Rapports et mémoires sur le sauvage de l'Aveyron.* Paris: Alcan.

JENKYN, L. and REEVES, A. (1979). Aphemia with hemiplegic migraine. *Neurology* **29**: 1317–1318.

JUDE and TRABAUD (1928). Hémiplégie gauche avec anarthrie. Accès de fou rire contrastant avec la correction de la mimique douloureuse. *Revue Neurologique* **2**: 726–728.

JÜRGENS, U. and VON CRAMON, D. (1982). On the role of the anterior cingulate cortex in phonation. A case report. *Brain and Language* **15**: 234–248.

KAAS, W., GILLMAN, A., MATTIS, S., KLUGMAN, E. and JACOBSON, B. (1967). Treatment of selective mutism in a blind child: School and clinic collaboration. *American Journal of Orthopsychiatry* **37**: 215–216.

KAHN, E., CROSLEY, E. and SCHNEIDER, R. (1969). *Correlative Neurosurgery.* Springfield, IL: Thomas.

KAPLAN, S. and ESCOLL, P. (1973). Treatment of two silent adolescent girls. *Journal of the American Academy of Child Psychiatry* **12**: 59–72.

KEITH, R. and ARONSON, A. (1975). Singing as therapy for apraxia of speech and aphasia: Report of a case. *Brain and Language* **2**: 483–488.

KLEE, A. (1961). Akinetic mutism: Review of the literature and report of a case. *Journal of Nervous and Mental Disease* **133**: 536–553.

KOHLER, C. and VUAGNAT, J. (1971). Mutisme et mutité. *Annales Médico-Psychologiques* **129**: 509–520.

KOLVIN, I. and FUNDUDIS, T. (1981). Electively mute children: Psychological development and background factors. *Journal of Child Psychology and Psychiatry* **22**: 219–232.

KROPPENBERG, D. (1987). Das dialogische Moment im menschlichen Spracherwerb mit einer kasuistischen Studie über dreizehnjährige eineiige Zwillinge mit selektivem Mutismus. In *Spracherwerb und Spracherwerbstörungen*, pp. 284–299. Hamburg: Wartenberg.

KUETTNER, W. (1959). Psychogene Aphonie als Massenerscheinung in einem Kinderheim. *Archiv für Ohren-, Nasen- und Kehlkopfheilkunde* **175**: 443–445.

KUPIETZ, S. and SCHWARTZ, I. (1982). Elective mutism. *New York State Journal of Medicine* **82**: 1073–1076.

LANE, H. (1977). *The Wild Boy of Aveyron*. London: Allen & Unwin.

LA RIVIERE, C., SEILO, M. and DIMMICK, K. (1975). Report on the speech intelligibility of a glossectomee: Perceptual and acoustic observations. *Folia Phoniatrica* **27**: 201–214.

LAUNAY, C. and BOREL-MAISONNY, S. (1972). *Les troubles du langage, de la parole et de la voix chez l'enfant*. Paris: Masson.

LAUNAY, C. and SOULE, M. (1952). Trois cas d'audio-mutité. *Archives Françaises de Pédiatrie* **1**: 754–759.

LEBRUN, Y. (1970). Clinical evidence against the motor theory of speech perception. In *Proceedings of the Sixth International Congress of Phonetic Sciences*, Prague, pp. 531–534.

LEBRUN, Y. (1973). *The Artificial Larynx*. Amsterdam-Lisse: Swets & Zeitlinger.

LEBRUN, Y. (1976). Neurolinguistic models of language and speech. In Whitaker, H. (Ed.) *Studies in Neurolinguistics 1*, pp. 1–30. New York: Academic Press.

LEBRUN, Y. (1978a). The inside of aphasia. In Lebrun, Y. and Hoops, R. (Eds) *The Management of Aphasia*, pp. 50–55. Lisse: Swets & Zeitlinger.

LEBRUN, Y. (1978b). Warum sprach Victor aus Aveyron nicht? *Zeitschrift für Kinder- und Jugendpsychiatrie* **6**: 396–408.

LEBRUN, Y. (1980). Victor of Aveyron. A reappraisal in light of more recent cases of feral speech. *Language Sciences* **2**: 32–43.

LEBRUN, Y. (1982). Aphasie de Broca et anarthrie. *Acta Neurologica Belgica* **82**: 80–90.

LEBRUN, Y. (1986). Aphasia with recurrent utterance: A review. *British Journal of Disorders of Communication* **21**: 3–10.

LEBRUN, Y. (1988a). Nuovi orientamenti nello studio dell'afasia acquisita nei bambini. *I Care* **13**: 77–80.

LEBRUN, Y. (1988b). Therapy-resistant dysarthria in a child. *Child Language and Therapy* **4**: 347–351.

LEBRUN, Y. (1989). Apraxia of speech: The history of a concept. In Square-Storer, P (Ed.) *Acquired Apraxia of Speech in Aphasic Adults*, pp. 3–19. London: Taylor & Francis.

LEBRUN, Y. and DEVREUX, F. (1984). Alexia in relation to aphasia and agnosia. In Malatesha, R. and Whitaker, H. (Eds) *Dyslexia: A global issue*, pp. 191–209. The Hague: Nijhoff.

LEBRUN, Y., DIERICK, M. and HOSSELAER, C. (1986). Disartria pseudobulbare acquisita in un bambino in eta scolare. *I Care* **11**: 128–131.

LENNEBERG, E. (1962). Understanding language without ability to speak: A case report. *Journal of Abnormal and Social Psychology* **65**: 419–425.

LENNEBERG, E. (1967). *Biological Foundations of Language*. New York: Wiley.

LESSER-KATZ, M. (1986). Stranger reaction and elective mutism in children. *American Journal of Orthopsychiatry* **56**: 458–469.

LEVIN, H. (1981). Aphasia in closed head injury. In Taylor Sarno, M. (Ed.) *Acquired Aphasia*, pp. 427–463. New York: Academic Press.

LEVIN, H., MADISON, C., BAILEY, C., MEYERS, C., EISENBERG, H. and GUINTO, F. (1983). Mutism after closed head injury. *Archives of Neurology* **40**: 601–606.

LEVINE, D. and MOHR, J. (1979). Language after bilateral cerebral infarctions: Role of the minor hemisphere in speech. *Neurology* **29**: 927–938.

LHERMITTE, F., GAUTIER, J.C., MARTEAU, R. and CHAIN, F. (1963). Troubles de la conscience et mutisme akinétique. *Revue Neurologique* **109**: 115–131.

LIBERMAN, A. (1957). Some results of research on speech perception. *Journal of the Acoustical Society of America* **29**: 117–123.

LIEBERMAN, A. and BENSON, D. (1977). Control of emotional expression in pseudo-bulbar palsy. *Archives of Neurology* **34**: 717–719.

LURIA, A. (1970). *Traumatic Aphasia.* The Hague: Mouton.

MARCOTTE, D. (1972). Marijuana and mutism. *American Journal of Psychiatry* **129**: 475–477.

MARIE, P. (1906a). La troisième circonvolution frontale gauche ne joue aucun rôle spécial dans la fonction du langage. *La Semaine Médicale* **26**: 241–247.

MARIE, P. (1906b). Que faut-il penser des aphasies sous-corticales? *La Semaine Médicale* **26**: 493–500.

MASDEU, J., SCHOENE, W. and FUNKENSTEIN, H. (1978). Aphasia following infarction of the left supplementary motor area. *Neurology* **28**: 1220–1223.

MASTERS, W., JOHNSON, V. and KOLODNY, R. (1986). *Masters and Johnson on Sex and Human Loving.* London: Macmillan.

MAURICE-WILLIAMS, R. (1972). Delayed akinetic mutism after subarachnoid haemorrhage. *Guy's Hospital Reports* **121**: 229–231.

MENDEL, K. (1912). Über Rechtshirnigkeit bei Rechtshändern. *Neurologisches Central-blatt* **31**: 156–165.

MENDEL, K. (1914). Über Rechtshirnigkeit bei Rechtshändern. *Neurologisches Central-latt* **33**: 291–293.

MESSERT, B., HENKE, T. and LANGHEIM, W. (1966). Syndrome of akinetic mutism associated with obstructive hydrocephalus. *Neurology* **16**: 635–649.

MORA, G., DEVAULT, S. and SCHOPLER, E. (1962). Dynamics and psychotherapy of identical twins with elective mutism. *Journal of Child Psychology and Psychiatry* **3**: 41–52.

MORGENSTERN, S. (1927). Un cas de mutisme psychogène. *Revue Française de Psychanalyse* **1**: 492–504.

MORIN, C., LADOUCEUR, R. and CLOUTIER, R. (1982). Reinforcement procedure in the treatment of reluctant speech. *Journal of Behavioural Therapy and of Experimental Psychiatry* **13**: 145–147.

MORRISH, E. (1988). Compensatory articulation in a subject with total glossectomy. *British Journal of Disorders of Communication* **23**: 13–22.

MUCK, O. (1917). Über Schnellheilungen von funktioneller Stummheit und Taubstummheit nebst einem Beitrag zur Kenntnis des Wesens des Mutismus. *Münchener medizinische Wochenschrift* **5**: 165–166.

MUNFORD, P., REARDON, D., LIBERMAN, R. and ALLEN, L. (1976). Behavioral treatment of hysterical coughing and mutism: A case study. *Journal of Consulting and Clinical Psychology* **44**: 1008–1014.

MURPHY, M., BRENTON, D., ASCHENBRENER, C. and VAN GILDER, J. (1979). Locked-in syndrome caused by a solitary pontine abscess. *Journal of Neurology, Neurosurgery and Psychiatry* **42**: 1062–1065.

MYQUEL, M. and GRANON, M. (1982). Le mutisme électif extrafamilial chez l'enfant. *Neuropsychiatrie de l'Enfance* **30**: 329–339.

NEBES, R. (1975). The nature of internal speech in a patient with aphemia. *Brain and Language* **2**: 489–497.

NIELSEN, J. (1951). Anterior cingulate gyrus and corpus callosum. *Bulletin of the Los Angeles Neurological Society* 16: 235–243.

NOLAN, C. (1981). *Dam-burst of Dreams.* London: Sphere Books.

NOLAN, C. (1987). *Under the Eye of the Clock.* London: Weidenfeld & Nicolson.

OJEMANN, G. (1976). Subcortical language mechanisms. In Whitaker, H. (Ed.) *Studies in Neurolinguistics 1*, pp. 103–138. New York: Academic Press.

PARTRIDGE, E. (1961). *A Dictionary of Slang and Unconventional English.* London: Routledge & Kegan Paul.

PELED, R., HARNES, B., BOROVICH, B. and SHARF, B. (1984). Speech arrest and supplementary motor area seizures. *Neurology* 34: 110–111.

PENFIELD, W. and JASPER, H. (1954). *Epilepsy and the Functional Anatomy of the Brain.* Boston: Little-Brown.

PENFIELD, W. and RASMUSSEN, T. (1949). Vocalization and arrest of speech. *Archives of Neurology* 61: 21–27.

PENFIELD, W. and ROBERTS, L. (1959). *Speech and Brain Mechanisms.* Princeton: Princeton University Press.

PENFIELD, W. and WELCH, K. (1951). The supplementary motor area of the cerebral cortex. *Archives of Neurology and Psychiatry* 66: 289–317.

PERTUISET, B. and PERRIER, F. (1960). Le syndrome operculaire unilatéral (rolandique inférieur) d'origine vasculaire. *Revue Neurologique* 103: 63–64.

PETIT-DUTAILLIS, D., GUIOT, G., MESSIMY, R. and BOURDILLON, C. (1954). A propos d'une aphémie par atteinte de la zone motrice supplémentaire de Penfield, au cours de l'évolution d'un anévrisme artério-veineux. Guérison de l'aphémie par ablation de la lésion. *Revue Neurologique* 90: 95–106.

PETTYGROVE, W. (1985). A psychosocial perspective on the glossectomy experience. *Journal of Speech and Hearing Research* 50: 107–109.

PIERRE-KAHN, A., MITJAVILLE, I., DEBRAY-RITZEN, P. and HIRSCH, J. (1980). Mutisme après chirurgie de la fosse postérieure chez l'enfant. *Revue Neurologique* 136: 92.

PUSTROM, E. and SPEERS, R. (1964). Elective mutism in children. *Journal of the American Academy of Child Psychiatry* 9: 287–297.

REED, G. (1963). Elective mutism in children: A re-appraisal. *Journal of Child Psychology and Psychiatry* 4: 99–107.

REID, J., HAWKINS, N., KEUTZER, C., MCNEAL, S., PHELPS, R., REID, K. and MEES, H. (1967). A marathon behaviour modification of a selectively mute child. *Journal of Child Psychology and Psychiatry* 8: 27–30.

REKATE, H., GRUBB, R., ARAM, D., HAHN, J. and RATCHESON, R. (1985). Muteness of cerebellar origin. *Archives of Neurology* 42: 697–698.

ROSENBAUM, E. and KELLMAN, M. (1973). Treatment of a selectively mute third-grade child. *Journal of School Psychology* 11. 26–29.

ROSENBERG, J. and LINDBLAD, M. (1978). Behavior therapy in a family context: Treating elective mutism. *Family Proceedings* 17: 77–81.

ROSS, E. and STEWART, M. (1981). Akinetic mutism from hypothalamic damage: Successful treatment with dopamine agonists. *Neurology* 31: 1435–1439.

RUFF, R. and ARBIT, E. (1981). Aphemia resulting from a left frontal hematoma. *Neurology* 31: 353–356.

RUGG, P. (1887). Aphonia: Recovery of a supposed 'incurable'. *British Medical Journal* July 9: 70.

RUSSELL, J. (1864). A case of hysteric aphonia. *British Medical Journal* 2: 619–621.

RUZICKA, B. and SACKIN, D. (1974). Elective mutism. *Journal of the American Academy of Child Psychiatry* 13: 551–561.

SCHACHTER, M. (1967). Aphémie suivie de bégaiement d'origine psychodramatique chez une fillette de 4 ans. *Acta Paedopsychiatrica* **34**: 13–17.

SCHACHTER, M. (1977). Le mutisme électif chez l'enfant d'âge préscolaire et scolaire. Contribution à la psychopathologie de la communication. *Schweizerischer Rundschau Medizin (Praxis)* **66**: 1442–1449.

SCOTT, E. (1977). A desensitization programme for the treatment of mutism in a seven year old girl: A case report. *Journal of Child Psychology and Psychiatry* **18**: 263–270.

SERDARU, M., LECHEVALIER, B. and GRAY, F. (1982). Encéphalopathie avec akinésie, myoclonies, troubles de la motricité d'un hémicorps et mutisme chez une femme d'âge moyen, alcoolique. *Revue Neurologique* **138**: 673–679.

SHARPE, E. (1940). Psycho-physical problems revealed in language: An examination of metaphor. *International Journal of Psychoanalysis* **21**: 201–213.

SHAW, W. (1971). Aversive control in the treatment of elective mutism. *Journal of the American Academy of Child Psychiatry* **10**: 572–581.

SHERMAN, J. (1963). Reinstatement of verbal behavior in a psychotic by reinforcement methods. *Journal of Speech and Hearing Disorders* **28**: 341–398.

SHERMAN, J. (1968). Use of reinforcement and imitation to reinstate verbal behavior in mute psychotics. In Sloane, H. and Macaulay, B. (Eds) *Operant Procedures in Remedial Speech and Language Training*, pp. 219–241. Boston: Houghton Mifflin.

SIMPSON, M., TILL, J. and GOFF, A. (1988). Long-term treatment of severe dysarthria: A case study. *Journal of Speech and Hearing Disorders* **53**: 433–440.

SKELLY, M., SPECTOR, D., DONALDSON, R., BRODEUR, A. and PALETTA, F. (1971). Compensatory physiologic phonetics for the glossectomee. *Journal of Speech and Hearing Disorders* **36**: 101–114.

SOUQUES, A. (1928). Quelques cas d'anarthrie de Pierre Marie. *Revue Neurologique* **2**: 319–368.

SMAYLING, L. (1959). Analysis of six cases of voluntary mutism. *Journal of Speech and Hearing Disorders* **24**: 55–58.

STARKSTEIN, S., BERTHIER, M. and LEIGUARDA, R. (1988). Bilateral opercular syndrome and crossed aphemia due to a right insular lesion: A clinicopathological study. *Brain and Language* **34**: 253–261.

STRAIT, R. (1958). A child who was speechless in school and social life. *Journal of Speech and Hearing Disorders* **23**: 253–254.

STRAUGHAN, J. (1968). The application of operant conditioning to the treatment of elective mutism. In Sloane, H. and Macaulay, B. (Eds) *Operant Procedures in Remedial Speech and Language Training*, pp. 242–258. Boston: Houghton Mifflin.

STRAUGHAN, J., POTTER, W. and HAMILTON, S. (1965). The behavioral treatment of an elective mute. *Journal of Child Psychology and Psychiatry* **6**: 125–130.

SUSSMAN, N., GUR, R., GUR, R. and O'CONNOR, M. (1983). Mutism as a consequence of callosotomy. *Journal of Neurosurgery* **59**: 514–519.

TODDROW, S. (1978). *Hirntrauma und Erlebnis.* Berne: Huber.

TOLENTINO, I. (1957). Inhibition du langage et mutisme en psychothérapie. *Acta Neurologica et Psychiatrica Belgica* **57**: 955–971.

TRAUT, E. (1935). The case of Patricia Maguire. *Journal of the American Medical Association* **104**: 1210–1212.

VALLAR, G. and CAPPA, S. (1987). Articulatory and verbal short-term memory: Evidence from anarthria. *Cognitive Neuropsychology* **4**: 55–78.

VAN BOGAERT, L. (1934). Ocular paroxysms and palilalia. *Journal of Nervous and Mental Disease* **80**: 48–61.

VAN HOUT, A. (1976). A case of long-standing mutism. In Lebrun, Y. and Hoops, R. (Eds) *Recovery in Aphasics*, pp. 230–234. Amsterdam: Swets & Zeitlinger.

VERNEA, J. (1974). Partial status epilepticus with speech arrest. *Proceedings of the Australian Association of Neurology* 11: 223–228.

VOLCAN, I., COLE, G. and JOHNSTON, K. (1986). A case of muteness of cerebellar origin. *Archives of Neurology* 34: 313–314.

WALLACE, M. (1987). *The Silent Twins*. London: Penguin.

WALLIS, H. (1957). Zur Systematik des Mutismus im Kindesalter. *Zeitschrift für Kinderpsychiatrie* 24: 129–133.

WASSING, H. (1973). A case of prolonged elective mutism in an adolescent boy: On the nature of the condition and its residential treatment. *Acta Paedopsychiatrica* 40: 75–96.

WERGELAND, H. (1979). Elective mutism. *Acta Psychiatrica Scandinavica* 59: 218–228.

WERNER, L. (1945). Treatment of a child with delayed speech. *Journal of Speech Disorders* 10: 329–334.

WRIGHT, H. (1968). A clinical study of children who refuse to talk in school. *Journal of the American Academy of Child Psychiatry* 7: 603–617.

WRIGHT, H., MILLER, D., COOK, M. and LITTMAN, J. (1985). Early identification and intervention with children who refuse to speak. *Journal of the American Academy of Child Psychiatry* 24: 739–746.

WUNDERLI, J. (1962). Ueber Anarthrie und Dysarthrie bei Parkinsonismus, infantiler Pseudobulbärparalyse und Schädeltrauma. *Schweizer Archiv für Neurologie, Neurochirurgie und Psychiatrie* 90: 74–103.

YOUNGERMAN, J. (1979). The syntax of silence: Electively mute therapy. *International Review of Psycho-Analysis* 6: 283–295.

ZELIGS, M. (1961). The psychology of silence. *Journal of the American Psychoanalytical Association* 9: 7–43.

Index (Author)

Abraham, 43, 49, 107
Adams, 56, 107
Ajuriaguerra, 47, 55, 107
Akhtar, 54, 107
Alajouanine, 74, 76, 77, 78, 79, 80, 107
Allen, 41, 112
Allende, 45
Altshuler, 1, 107
Aram, 96, 113
Arbit, 84, 113
Arnold, 57, 107
Aronson, 103, 110
Arts, 70, 107
Augustine (St), 8

Babinski, 2, 97, 107
Bach, 52, 107
Bacon, 6
Bailey, 85, 86, 87, 112
Bak, 70, 107
Barris, 98, 107
Barton, 62, 107
Basso, 44, 107
Bauermeister, 29, 35, 108
Bednar, 17, 18, 38, 108
Benedict (St), 7
Benson, 46, 60, 61, 81, 109, 112
Benton, 103, 108
Berthier, 76, 77, 78, 79, 80, 108, 114
Bittorf, 52, 53, 108
Blotcky, 42, 108
Boetius, 5
Bogen, 97, 108
Bone, 84, 109
Borel-Maisonny, 57, 111

Borovich, 99, 113
Botez, 99, 101, 108
Boucharlat, 75, 108
Boudin, 79, 107
Bourdillon, 78, 80, 100, 113
Bradley, 25, 108
Brage, 96, 108
Broca, 80, 108
Brodeur, 64, 114
Brown, 48, 52, 108
Buckman, 54, 107
Buge, 90, 108

Cairns, 90, 91, 94, 96, 108
Cambier, 76, 77, 78, 80, 107
Campion, 5
Cappa, 75, 88, 102, 108, 114
Carbonell, 47, 109
Carlyle, 6
Chain, 91, 96, 112
Chateau, 75, 108
Chatelain, 75, 108
Chethik, 20, 43, 46, 108
Chia, 76, 77, 78, 108
Chopler, 18, 22, 23, 26, 30, 31, 112
Cicero, 7
Cloutier, 19, 29, 112
Cohen, 29, 32, 110
Cole, 96, 115
Colligan, 28, 109
Cook, 19, 20, 34, 42, 115
Copello, 96, 108
Critchley, 38, 50, 109
Cronin, 36
Crosley, 89, 110

117

Cummings, 1, 46, 60, 61, 107, 109

Dalin, 103
Daly, 94, 96, 109
Damasio, 76, 77, 78, 109
D'Ambrosio, 42, 49, 55, 109
David, 84, 109
De Bruine Groeneveldt, 62, 109
De Gobineau, 47, 107
De Mol, 85, 109
De Morsier, 84, 109
Debray-Ritzen, 95, 96, 113
Dejerine, 103, 109
Deleval, 85, 109
Denes, 102, 109
Devault, 18, 22, 23, 26, 30, 31, 112
Devreux, 2, 11
Diatkine, 47, 107
Dierick, 70, 111
Dillard, 28, 109
Dimmick, 64, 111
Doms, 71, 109
Donaldson, 64, 114
Dugas, 47, 109
Dumas, 89
Dumond, 41, 43, 50, 109

Eisenberg, 85, 86, 87, 112
Elliott, 68, 109
Elson, 18, 22, 109
Escoll, 23, 42, 48, 110
Escourolle, 90, 108

Fau, 75, 108
Fourcin, 66, 109
Fundudis, 19, 20, 22, 24, 34, 35, 42, 111
Funkenstein, 84, 112

Gargan, 62, 109
Garoux, 41, 43, 50, 109
Gauger, 88, 109
Gautier, 91, 96, 112
Gersh, 76, 77, 78, 109
Gilmore, 99, 109
Glassner, 56, 107
Goff, 89, 114
Goldiamond, 53, 110
Goldstein, 64, 109
Goll, 19, 20, 21, 23, 25, 27, 38, 42, 47, 109
Gosenfeld, 46, 60, 61, 109

Gouaze, 95, 110
Granon, 18, 19, 24, 35, 37, 112
Gray, 95, 114
Grimm, 6, 10
Groslambert, 75, 108
Grosswasser, 72, 110
Grosswasser-Reider, 72, 110
Grotjahn, 90, 96, 110
Grubb, 96, 113
Gueriot, 47, 109
Guidetti, 99, 100, 110
Guidotti, 75, 108
Guinto, 85, 86, 87, 112
Guiot, 78, 80, 100, 113
Gur, 98, 114
Guttman, 86, 110

Hahn, 96, 113
Halpern, 29, 32, 110
Hamilton, 17, 29, 33, 35, 114
Hammond, 29, 32, 110
Harnes, 99, 113
Hawkins, 28, 30, 113
Hayakawa, 40, 110
Hayden, 17, 50, 110
Head, 78, 110
Heilman, 99, 109
Henke, 93, 94, 96, 112
Herodotus, 53
Hill, 20, 21, 35, 110
Hirsch, 95, 96, 113
Hirschfeld, 52, 53, 110
Hosselaer, 70, 111
Houlihan, 46, 60, 61, 109
Hughlings Jackson, 97

Inbody, 94, 110
Irving, 64
Issacs, 53, 110
Itard, 67, 110

Jankovic, 94, 110
Jarkowski, 97, 107
Jasper, 94, 113
Jemail, 29, 35, 108
Jenkyn, 99, 110
Johnson, 43, 112
Johnston, 96, 115
Jones, 18, 22, 109
Joynt, 103, 108

Jude, 75, 76, 77, 78, 80, 110
Jürgens, 90, 91, 110

Kahn, 89, 110
Kaplan, 23, 42, 48, 110
Keith, 103, 110
Kellman, 27, 113
Keutzer, 28, 30, 113
Kinsbourne, 76, 77, 78, 108
Klee, 90, 91, 94, 110
Kohler, 47, 111
Kolodny, 43, 112
Kolvin, 19, 20, 22, 24, 34, 35, 111
Korn, 72, 110
Kroppenberg, 23, 111
Kupietz, 18, 28, 35, 111

La Riviere, 64, 111
Ladouceur, 19, 29, 112
Lane, 67, 111
Langheim, 93, 94, 96, 112
Launay, 34, 57, 111
Lawrence, 39
Lebatard, 95, 110
Lebrun, 2, 63, 68, 70, 71, 84, 86, 88, 99,
    101, 102, 103, 106, 111
Lechevalier, 95, 114
Lefebvre, 76, 77, 78, 80, 107
Léger, 41, 43, 50, 109
Leiguarda, 76, 77, 78, 79, 80, 108, 114
Lenneberg, 67, 68, 111
Lesser-Katz, 24, 111
Levin, 85, 86, 87, 111, 112
Lhermitte, 76, 77, 78, 80, 91, 96, 107
Liberman A., 102, 112
Liberman R., 41, 112
Lieberman, 81, 112
Lindblad, 33, 113
Littman, 19, 20, 34, 42, 115
Llewellyn-Jones, 43, 49, 107
Lombartie, 41, 43, 50, 109
Looney, 42, 108
Love, 94, 96, 109
Luria, 49, 112

McNeil, 28, 30, 113
Madison, 85, 86, 87, 112
Magnus, 74
Malauzat, 41, 43, 50, 109
Marcotte, 100, 112

Marie, 77, 78, 81, 112
Marteau, 91, 96, 112
Masdeu, 84, 112
Masters, 43, 112
Mees, 28, 30, 113
Mendel, 76, 77, 78, 81, 112
Messert, 93, 94, 96, 112
Messimy, 78, 80, 100, 113
Meyers, 85, 86, 87, 112
Miller, 19, 20, 34, 42, 115
Mills, 1, 107
Mitjaville, 95, 96, 113
Mora, 18, 22, 23, 26, 30, 31, 112
Morea, 96, 108
Morgenstein, 44, 47, 51, 112
Morin, 19, 29, 112
Morrish, 64, 112
Muck, 52, 53, 112
Munford, 41, 112
Myquel, 18, 19, 24, 35, 37, 112

Nebes, 102, 112
Needleman, 68, 109
Nielsen, 93, 113
Nolan, 66, 113

O'Connor, 98, 114
Ojemann, 100, 113
Oldfield, 90, 91, 94, 96, 108
Ovid, 40

Paletta, 64, 114
Papagno, 75, 108
Partridge, 44, 113
Pearson, 18, 22, 109
Peled, 99, 113
Penfield, 94, 100, 113
Pennybacker, 90, 91, 94, 96, 108
Pépin, 79, 107
Perret, 75, 108
Perrier, 79, 113
Pertruiset, 79, 107, 113
Petit-Dutaillis, 77, 80, 100, 113
Pettygrove, 64, 113
Phelps, 28, 30, 113
Pierre-Kahn, 95, 96, 113
Plichet, 97, 107
Poisson, 90, 108
Potter, 17, 29, 33, 35, 114
Prirovano, 88, 108

Pustrom, 17, 20, 21, 22, 23, 24, 30, 42, 113

Rancurel, 90, 108
Rasmussen, 100, 113
Ratcheson, 96, 113
Reardon, 41, 112
Reed, 32, 35, 113
Reeves, 99, 110
Reid, 28, 30, 113
Rekate, 96, 113
Rizzo, 76, 77, 78, 109
Roberts, 100, 113
Rolland, 95, 110
Rondat, 76, 77, 78, 80, 107
Rosenbraun, 27, 113
Rosenberg, 33, 113
Ross, 94, 113
Ruff, 84, 113
Rugg, 47, 50, 113
Russell, 42, 43, 113
Ruzicka, 17, 26, 113

Sackin, 17, 26, 113
Schachter, 19, 20, 38, 47, 114
Schneider, 89, 110
Schoene, 84, 112
Schönberg, 8
Schumacher, 18, 22, 109
Schuman, 98, 107
Schwartz, 18, 28, 35, 111
Scott, 17, 18, 23, 32, 114
Scull, 20, 21, 35, 110
Seilo, 64, 111
Serdaru, 95, 114
Sharf, 99, 113
Sharpe, 21, 114
Shaw, 19, 25, 29, 38, 114
Sherman, 54, 114
Simenon, 36, 39, 40
Simpson, 89, 114
Skelly, 64, 114
Sloman, 25, 108
Smayling, 35, 69, 114
Solzi, 72, 110
Soulé, 34, 111
Souques, 76, 77, 78, 81, 97, 114

Spector, 64, 114
Speers, 17, 20, 21, 22, 23, 24, 30, 42, 113
Starkstein, 76, 77, 78, 79, 80, 108, 114
Stewart, 94, 113
Strait, 16, 17, 38, 114
Straughan, 17, 26, 29, 33, 35, 47, 114
Sussman, 98, 114
Swinburne, 6

Thomas, 53, 110
Thurel, 74, 107
Till, 89, 114
Todorow, 86, 114
Tolentino, 37, 49, 50, 114
Trabaud, 75, 76, 77, 78, 81, 110
Traut, 95, 114

Valéry, 6
Vallar, 88, 102, 114
Van Bogaert, 96, 114
Van Dongen, 70, 107
Van Hout, 71, 114
Varney, 76, 77, 78, 109
Velin, 47, 109
Vercors, 7
Vernea, 98, 115
Vignolo, 75, 88, 108
Vigny, 6
Volcan, 96, 115
Vogel, 97, 108
Von Cramon, 90, 91, 110
Vuagnat, 47, 111

Wallace, 19, 25, 40, 42, 115
Wallis, 51, 115
Wassing, 17, 18, 20, 32, 115
Welch, 100, 113
Wergeland, 19, 20, 25, 30, 31, 34, 115
Werner, 55, 115
Wertheim, 99, 108
Whitteridge, 90, 91, 94, 96, 108
Wlatt, 79, 108
Wright, 19, 20, 24, 34, 42, 115
Wunderli, 97, 115

Youngerman, 19, 23, 26, 42, 115

Zeligs, 38, 115

Index (Subject)

Aaron, 8
Abulia, 86
acquired mutism, 61, 69–104
affect, 53, 93, 96, 97
agenesis of the tongue, 64
aggressiveness, 38, 50, 51
akinesia, 86, 90, 93, 94, 96
akinetic mutism, 61, 89–95
amimia, *see* facial expression
amyotrophic lateral sclerosis, 81
anarthria, 68, 81
ankyloglossia, 64
anorexia, 42, 43
apallism, 92–93
apathy, 86
aphasia, 48
aphasia with recurrent utterance, 88
aphasic mutism, 83–88, 100
aphemia, 80
aphonia, 46–47
    see also whispering
apraxia, 80, 93, 94, 103
    see also oral apraxia; speech apraxia
articulation in the glossectomees, 64
artificial larynx, 63
assertiveness, 38, 48, 57
audio-mutitas, 67
autism, 61
automatic–voluntary dissociation, 73, 74, 75, 79, 80
aversive stimulus, 29–30
avolition, 91

behaviour modification, 26–30, 32, 33, 41, 53, 54
Bible, 5, 6, 7, 8, 9, 39, 44

bi-opercular syndrome, *see* opercular syndrome
Boydell, 66, 68
breath, 37
Broca's aphasia, 81, 103
bulbar mutism, 82
bulbar palsy, 81–82

castration, 45, 51
catatonia, 53, 55, 90, 93
cerebellum, 96
cerebral palsy, 65–66, 82
chewing difficulties, *see* dysphagia
classroom mutism, 17, 28, 29
clinical–semiological approach, 1–2
coma vigil, 92
congenital malformations of the vocal tract, 64
congenital motor aphasia, *see* developmental motor aphasia
copulating, *see* making love
cortical motor aphasia, 81, 103
coughing, 41, 52
Croesus, 53

de-afferented state, *see* locked-in syndrome
deaf–muteness, 64–65
deafness, 48, 57
defaecation, 45
    see also toileting
developmental motor aphasia, 67–68
developmental mutism, 61, 65–69
developmental speech apraxia, 68–69
diaschisis, 98, 104

drawing, 51, 57, 97
dumbness, 9, 10
dysarthria, 70, 75, 78, 79, 83, 84, 87, 96
dysphagia, 70, 71, 72, 73, 74, 75, 76, 80,
    82, 84, 96

eating, 42–43, 44, 45, 46, 90
eating problems, 42, 60, 97
    see also dysphagia
elective mutism, see selective mutism
electric current, 52
emotional lability, see spasmodic laughing
encopresis, 20–21, 45, 47
enuresis, 20–21, 45, 47
extrafamilial mutism, 17, 25, 28, 29, 34,
    35, 37, 42
eye contact, 18
epilepsy, see seizures

facial expression, 16, 17, 46, 51, 60, 73,
    74, 75, 76, 90
facio-labio-linguopharyngeal palsy, see
    opercular syndrome
familial isolation, 25–26
familial secret, 24
flaccid facial diplegia, see opercular
    syndrome
Foix–Chavany–Marie syndrome, see
    opercular syndrome
fright, 20, 52, 53
functional mutism, 1, 12, 13, 14–58,
    60–61, 86, 87, 105
    see also selective mutism; total mutism
functional paralysis, 48

global aphasia, 88, 92, 93
glossectomy, 63–64
God, 7, 8

hepatolenticular degeneration, 82
Hörstummheit, 67
hyperkinetic mutism, 94–95
hypnosis, 27, 52
hysterical mutism, 13, 41, 48, 75
    see also total mutism

incontinence, 90
    see also enuresis; encopresis
infantile pseudobulbar mutism, see
    infantile supranuclear mutism
infantile supranuclear mutism, 66

involuntary mutism, 2, 3, 9, 10, 12

Jesus, 6, 8, 9

Larbaud, 105
laryngectomees, 62
laryngectomy, 62
larynx, 43, 52, 53
lenticular zone, 78
lip-reading, 65
literary examples, 1
locked-in syndrome, 88–89, 93
love, 39, 40, 43, 44
    see also making love

making love, 39, 40, 44, 45, 46
    see also love
masturbation, 45
menstruation, 43
mirror-writing, 76
monastery, 7–8
Monte Cristo syndrome, see locked-in
    syndrome
morse code, 81, 88
Moses, 8
motor theory of speech perception, 102–
    103
mothers of selective mutes, 21, 22, 30
motor aphasia, 81, 83, 87, 103
motor neurone, 81
motor neurone disease, 81, 82
mouth, 37, 38, 39, 42, 43, 97
multiple sclerosis, 82
mutism
    associated with a pyramidal
        hemisyndrome, 61, 75–81
    after commissurotomy, 97–98
    definition of, 1, 11
    in parkinsonism, 96–97
    of peripheral origin, 62–65
    after surgery in the fossa posterior,
        95–96
    see also akinetic mutism; aphasic
        mutism; bulbar mutism;
        developmental mutism; functional
        mutism; hyperkinetic mutism;
        hysterical mutism; infantile
        supranuclear mutism; opercular
        mutism; organic mutism;
        paradoxical mutism; pseudobulbar

mutism, (cont.)
    mutism; selective mutism; total
    mutism
myasthenia gravis, 82

Nolan, 66, 68
non-verbal communication, see silent
    communication

oesophageal speech, 63
operant conditioning, see behaviour
    modification
opercular mutism, 81
opercular syndrome, 73–75, 78, 79, 80
operculum frontoparietalis, see
    operculum Rolandi
operculum Rolandi, 73, 74, 75, 84
oral apraxia, 80, 98
organic mutism, 12, 13, 59–104, 105, 106

palilalia, 12
panic, 12
paradoxical mutism, 97
parents of mute children, 22, 23, 33, 34,
    51
parkinsonism, 96–97
Pierre Marie's quadrilateral, 78
pseudobulbar mutism, 70–73, 81
pseudobulbar palsy, 69–73, 78, 79, 80, 81
psychodynamic procedures, see
    psychotherapy
psychogenic mutism, see functional
    mutism
psychosis, 54, 55
psychotherapy, 30–33, 41, 51, 57
pure motor aphasia, 81, 103
pyramidal hemisyndrome, see mutism
    associated with a pyramidal
    hemisyndrome

reluctant speech, 18–19, 29, 48
reticence, see reluctant speech

schizophrenia, 53–55, 58
school mutism, 17
Scriptures, see Bible
seizures, 84, 96, 97, 98, 99

selective mutism, 15–40, 45, 47, 49, 58
    in children with language delay, 34–35,
        69
    in children with normal command of
        language, 16–34
    definition of, 16
    dynamics of, 21–22
    eating problems in, 42
    as a family problem, 23–24
    in immigrant families, 25
    late onset of speech in, 35–36
    mental handicap in, 35, 37
    reactions of the environment to, 26, 31
    sex ratio in, 19–20
    spontaneous recovery from, 34
    therapy for, 26–34
self-exposure, 38
semiotics, 2
semi-voluntary mutism, 2, 12
separation difficulties, 22
sex-bound mutism, 17
sexual intercourse, see making love
sialorrhoea, 70, 80, 97
silence, 5–10, 57, 105
silent communication, 18, 19, 50, 57
singing, 103
soul kiss, 38
spasmodic laughter and spasmodic
    weeping, 70, 76, 79, 81
speaking, 20, 21, 37, 39, 40, 43, 44, 45, 46
speech, see speaking
speech apraxia, 101–104
    see also developmental speech apraxia
speech arrests, 98–101
    caused by electrical stimulation,
        99–100
    in catalepsy, 100
    due to intoxication, 100
    in epilepsy, 98–99
    migrainous, 99
    in narcolepsy, 101
speech therapy, 34, 35, 56, 57, 69, 70, 71,
    72, 83, 87, 89, 95, 97
stage fright, 12
stimulus-fading programme, 28
stuttering, 47–50
subcortical motor aphasia, 81
suggestion, 51
supplementary motor area, 78, 100

swallowing difficulties, *see* dysphagia
syndrome of the Sleeping Beauty, 86–87

talkativeness, 6, 44
throat, 41, 42, 43
toileting, 20, 21, 45, 46
total aphasia, *see* global aphasia
total mutism, 41–58
   in battle field casualties, 48–49, 50, 52
   dynamics of, 49–59
   in individuals with normal language
      development, 41–55
   in individuals with underdeveloped
      language skills, 55–57
   onset of, 46–47
   prognosis of, 50
   in psychotics, 54–55
   recovery from, 50, 52
   in schizophrenics, 53–55
   therapy for, 50–53
   throat infections in, 41–42

twins, 18, 19, 22, 23, 26, 30, 31, 40, 42

urination, 45
   see also toileting

vagina, 39, 45
ventral pontine state, *see* locked-in
   syndrome
Versailles, 45
Victor of Aveyron, 67–68
voluntary mutism, 2, 11, 12

Western Apaches, 44
whispering, 19, 30, 32, 33, 47, 50, 84, 85,
   86, 90, 91, 98
Wilson's disease, *see* hepatolenticular
   degeneration
writing, 11, 30, 37, 40, 47, 51, 57, 68, 70,
   71, 73, 75, 76, 81, 84, 85, 97, 98, 99,
   101
written language, *see* writing